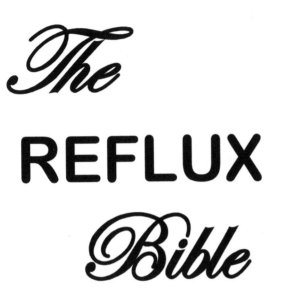

REFLUX

Second Edition 2015

Cherie Bacon Byrne

Copyright © 2015 by Cherie Bacon Byrne

Published by Cherie Bacon Byrne

Email: **TheRefluxBible@Gmail.Com**

Web: **www.TheRefluxBible.com**

ISBN 13: (Paperback) 978-0-9933416-0-1

Editing by Dr Jennifer Conlan BA (Mod Physiol.) MB, BCh, BAO MSc

Editing by **Karen O' Hanlon Cohrt, PH.D**

Editing by **Antonia Corrigan (M.B.S., M.I.I.E., Dip. Food Sc., Dip. App. Biol.)**

Cover Designed by **Orla O'Connor @ www.allindesign.ie**

Contents

Chapter 16 _____ 218

GORD and Emotions - The Personal Side __ 218

Tables & Figures

About the Author

Cherie Bacon Byrne was born and reared on Dublin city's north side.

Her previous working background prior to having her third baby, Raven, was predominantly within social care.

Cherie worked for six years in various social care settings, mostly as a high support youth worker. She worked with young people in residential care units and young persons in out-of-home placements and was highly respected amongst her peers. She was also a youth advocate trainer on the west coast of Ireland.

Cherie soon found her niche was working with young mothers and their babies. Mentoring her clients, guiding them in caring for their babies, and advising them on how to manage everyday living as new mums was a thoroughly enjoyable experience for her. In addition, Cherie worked in mother and baby units and did outreach work. She also conducted supervised access visits with clients and their families.

In 2011 she married her husband Lee and they decided to have a baby together. Cherie was, at that time, already a mother of two teenage children. On the 20th of November 2012, Raven Juliet Bacon Byrne came into their lives and the mayhem began.

The insatiable screams due to Raven's pain rang out in their home for many months to follow. Frustration and despair were the everyday reality of her family. Cherie describes this time in her life to resembling hell on earth.

The struggle to find a diagnosis and to be able to ease the obvious pain Raven was in was well and truly under way. The lack of understanding of the constant distress and daily challenges from not only the professionals involved in Ravens early years, but also from family and friends, was a very isolating experience.

The complete lack of understanding, formal knowledge or support, regarding the disease itself and the traumatic impact it had on Cherie and her family, inspired her to write her book *The Reflux Bible*.

The book is an attempt to share the knowledge gained and the war fought to find a source of information and explanation as to why their baby was in such distress from the beginning. Hopefully it will inform and support other mothers and families struggling with this illness and offer some hope that help can be found and that babies will enjoy a normal life.

The Second Edition of the Reflux Bible is Dedicated to my Second Mother

Ann Fagan R.I.P.

24th December 1936

To

9th February 2014

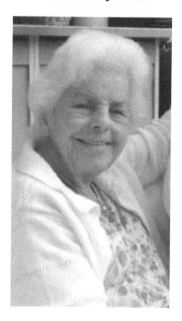

Gone but never forgotten

Acknowledgments

Reflux Disease is such an isolating illness. It is nearly impossible to have visitors, or indeed anyone, help with normal baby-minding jobs as life with this is far from normal. The virtually constant baby screaming and apparent distress is terrifying for anyone involved in your life. Distressed, embarrassed and desperate to find a way to help my baby, I shut myself off from the outside world.

I would like to acknowledge and thank my friends and family for all the support I received in writing my book.

To my good friend Evelyn Hannan, who tried to be there for me and called many times to our home but I just couldn't face anyone. I felt it was impossible to pretend to feel any kind of normal while my baby Raven was in such obvious pain and distress.

To my parents, now in their seventies, who have always given me a fair share of support with my children, over the years. However, in Raven's case I was afraid and uncomfortable to leave her with them, as she was in such distress constantly, and the fear and distress spread to everyone around her.

To my husband's family who assisted when they could. They minded Raven and were reassuringly confident with her, even at her worst. I cannot thank you enough for being there for her and for me when we needed help most, something I will always be grateful for.

To my sister Maria, who is brilliant with Raven, particularly now that she is that bit older and not so scary to mind!

To my husband Lee Byrne, who is amazing and was patient with both Raven and me. Reflux disease can destroy the strongest of marriages. We have had serious ups and downs and our love has been tested without a doubt, but we have hung in there and I'm in no doubt that better times will come and this experience will stand to us.

To my two older children Feile and Ryan, who have also lived this rollercoaster ride, I would never have been able to do all this without their support.

Feile had taken something of a back seat within the family since Raven came along. The understanding and support she has given me has been remarkable for a teenage girl. She would go to school in the mornings with Raven screaming and return to the same scenario every single day. She was visibly exhausted from being kept awake all night from Raven's screaming. At one stage, Feile had a breakdown in school; she simply could not take any more. She would frequently tell me she could hear Raven screaming in her mind, even when she wasn't around. The sound of her screams was like a constant fire alarm going off in our home for months. Feile, I thank you for your patience and kindness and how amazing you are with Raven and how well you did in your exams despite all that was going on at home.

To my lifelong friend Yvonne Wall, who stayed with me through thick and thin and held me up when I couldn't go on, even though she has her own silent reflux child with ASD. She was and is my rock and I will forever be indebted to her. I wish to thank my good friend and ally, Hazel Ahern in helping edit my book, listen to me whinging, and spurring me on.

Thank you also to Dr Jennifer Conlan BA (Mod Physiol.) MB, BCh, BAO MSc, who has reviewed and endorsed all medical information contained within this book.

Thanks also to Antonia Corrigan, my mentor and friend who helped me so much with this second edition. To Karen O' Hanlon Cohrt, Ph.D, who did the final edits of this book.

To all the authors, websites and associations that so kindly permitted me to directly use excerpts from their research, I thank you. This book is about putting all the research and medical information in one easy accessible place for parents surviving reflux. I have chosen excerpts that I have found useful in my search for answers. This book mainly consists of this information, peppered with my own story and voices of other parents struggling with this disease.

I also wish to thank Our Lady's Hospital, Crumlin in Dublin, especially our paediatrician who thoroughly helped Raven and all of us as a family. We found the hospital staff and specialist expertise in this hospital to be second to none. They literally saved my sanity and restored our faith in the medical profession.

And finally to my support group of wonderful warriors, the amazing resilient women of Surviving Reflux Ireland (SRI), who kept me sane and kept me going through all of this. The passion I have for the group is held dearly within my heart.

I also wish to thank my fabulous administrator, friend, sister, partner, Monica Brogan. I met Monica through the group over 2 years ago. We have a great bond and mutual admiration for each other, we hold each other up so we can in turn hold up others. Monica I thank you from the bottom of my heart for your support and time you have devoted in helping me with this book. I will look forward to ventures with you in the future.

This book is dedicated to all the members of SRI (Surviving Reflux Ireland). I have included many views, experiences and stories that the group members have kindly shared with me.

While every effort has been made to ensure the accuracy of the content of this book, I feel that a disclaimer is merited here, as I don't wish to get my ass sued!! Any suggestions or information is from my own personal experience and the experience of others. It is not intended to replace any medical professional. Always consult your doctor for medical advice and treatment.

You will notice as you read this book that I have used, for the most part, the European spelling for many of the medical terms, as distinct from the US spellings. Example; oesophagus (Eur.), esophagus (US) or behaviour (Eur.) and behaviour (US). Both have been used to reflect the original sources of the references and information.

Introduction

Here is My Story Here is My Heart

Raven Juliet was born in November 2012 with bilateral talipes[1], also known as clubfoot. Raven was soon diagnosed with significant gastro-oesophageal reflux disease (GORD) at three weeks old. She also developed severe feeding issues and had numerous food intolerances.

She started Ponseti treatment[2] for her talipes at three days old. This consisted of both her feet being manipulated and put into casts. Although this treatment is considered non-invasive, Raven could not tolerate the casts at all and was in constant distress. This condition coupled with silent reflux was hell for us as a family. Raven is my third child and my second reflux baby.

---

[1] Miedzybrodzka, Z (January 2003). *Congenital talipes equinovarus (clubfoot): a disorder of the foot but not the hand. .Journal of anatomy* **202** (1): 37–42. PMID 12587918.

[2] Patient Education Institute, *Treating club foot with Ponseti Treatment,* www.nlm.nih.gov/medlineplus/tutorials/treatingclubfoot/op [Accessed Jan 2015]

Normal baby soothing methods did not work for us and we made many a frantic dash to A&E. Raven developed laryngomalacia[3] and a stridor resulting from her silent reflux when she was three months old (see chapter 13 for explanations of common problems caused by GORD). She would stop breathing for episodes and vomit in her sleep through the night. I walked the floor with Raven day and night for what seemed like an eternity. The next 30 months of her life were to be the hardest challenge I have ever had to endure.

No one seemed to have any answers and doctors were baffled as to why she was in such distress. She screamed like a baby withdrawing from crack cocaine from morning to night. I trawled through the internet night after night looking for answers. No one seemed to understand. Only small groups of online support in the UK and the USA held any answers. I couldn't find one single place for information on this condition in Ireland, which is what spurred me to set up my support group "*Surviving Reflux Ireland.*"

This book is my way of giving back everything I have had to learn and to connect with parents suffering through this awful, baffling, and lonely disease.

---

[3] Lovinsky-Desir, Stephanie MD, Laryngomalacia-Medescape-Reference [Online] Available at: emedicine.medscape.com/article/1002527-overview, 28 Mar 2014

This book is based on the stories of Irish mothers, medical information and references. Advice on products, services and procedures and everything there is to know about reflux from a parent's perspective is also presented.

Chapter 1

What is Reflux[4]?

"Gastro-oesophageal reflux (GOR) is the passage of gastric contents into the oesophagus. It is considered physiological in infants when symptoms are absent or not troublesome.

Gastro-oesophageal reflux disease (GORD) in children is the presence of troublesome symptoms or complications arising from GOR.

GOR occurs as a result of transient lower oesophageal sphincter (LES) muscle relaxation. Several anatomical and physiological features (such as delayed gastric emptying and short, narrow oesophagus) make infants (younger than one year old) more prone to GOR than older children and adults. GOR and GORD may also be caused by cow's milk protein allergy.

---

[4] National Institute for Health and Care Excellence, *Gastro-oesophageal reflux disease: recognition, diagnosis and management in children and young people,* 2014 Available at http://nice.org.uk/.../**gord**-in-children-guideline-consultation-draft-**nice**-gord-in-children-guideline-consultation-draft-nice-guideline2 [Accessed July 2014]

Most children have no specific risk factors for GORD. However, children with certain conditions (such as cystic fibrosis, severe neurological impairment, and gastro-oesophageal abnormalities) are at an increased risk of developing GORD.

Complications that may occur in children with GORD include anaemia, chronic cough, and wheezing. GORD improves with age and can usually be diagnosed clinically. GORD should be suspected in children with either (but usually both) of the following:

1. *Frequent and troublesome regurgitation or vomiting (which may occur up to two hours after feeding).*
2. *Frequent and troublesome crying, irritability, or back-arching during or after feeding, food refusal (despite being willing to suck on a dummy).*

Children with GORD may also have oesophageal symptoms such as anaemia and dysphasia, respiratory symptoms such as asthma or reactive airways disease, and other symptoms such as sleeping difficulties and dental erosion".

It is said that reflux mainly starts at six weeks old and peaks at four months. Reflux that persists and needs medication is known as GORD. GORD can continue right into the toddler stage of development and may need ongoing medical care and investigations. Please see Diagram & illustrations of the anatomy of a baby which is shown in figure 1 below.

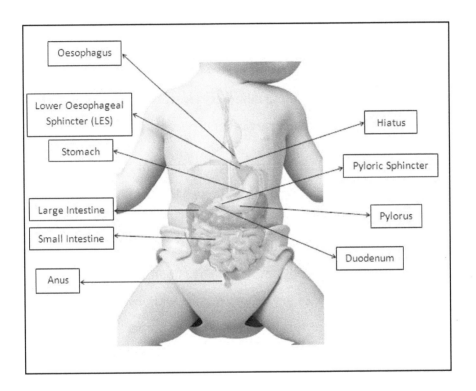

Figure 1: Diagram & Illustrations of the Anatomy of a Baby

Distinguishing Between GOR & GORD

Reflux can occur along a severity continuum, ranging from mild reflux, Known as 'GOR' (gastro-oesophageal reflux), to the more severe type known as gastro-oesophageal reflux disease 'GORD'. Although similar in many ways, there are a number of important differences between the two states, and recognizing these differences is crucial in both managing reflux and in finding the correct medication if necessary.

GOR can correct itself when a baby is roughly three or four months old and can usually be effectively managed through lifestyle changes such as adding a thickener to feeds, avoiding overfeeding, holding the child in the upright position for 30 minutes. This kind of reflux is tough going. I can still remember the constant screaming, floor walking and poor feeding, as well as a lack of any proper routine with my first child who had GOR. Nevertheless, it rectified itself when he turned three months old.

GORD, however, is totally different. The severities of the attacks are much worse and prolonged.

With GORD, normal coping mechanisms and the management techniques, such as keeping the baby upright after feeds, using stay down formula etc, will not work. Medication is almost always needed and the child can display symptoms for well over a year and in some instances, a lot longer. GORD is a long term illness, a disease; the child will need ongoing medical care and investigations. It can also cause a multitude of other health problems.

This information is crucial for any parent or caregiver dealing with this problem. Unfortunately GOR and GORD get thrown into the one pot that is called "Reflux." This is extremely frustrating for parents, as it is like comparing the common cold to pneumonia.

Parents and children struggle with this awful disease, often lacking support and understanding from surroundings, not least the medical profession. The majority of family members and friends and the wider community in general are completely unaware that there is a difference between reflux (GOR) and reflux disease (GORD). Many people are not even aware of reflux in the first place. I now tell people Raven has reflux disease or GORD. It saves me from hearing a lot of the preconceptions that people may have about the disease and it lets them know that there is certainly a huge difference in the pain of the baby and the struggles of the parents.

Symptoms of Colic[5]

"About 40 years ago, a paediatrician named Dr. Morris Wessel conducted a breakthrough study on excessively fussy children. The definition he chose to use to describe colicky babies was not considered scientific, but it stuck with physicians. His definition of a colicky infant was a child who cried for more than 3 hours a day, for more than 3 days a week, for over 3 weeks. This is often referred to as the "Rule of 3's" and these rules came to be known as the Wessel Criteria[6], which is now used in most current studies of babies with colic".

---

[5] American Pregnancy Association, 2014. *Colic.* [Online] Available at:
http://americanpregnancy.org/first-year-of-life/colic/
[Accessed 15 May 2014].

[6] Wessel MA, et al. *Rule of three: Paroxismal fussing in infancy, sometimes called "colic."* Pediatrics. 1954; 14:421-435. Quoted in *Birth & beyond/ Colic*, American Pregnancy Association Available at http://americanpregnancy.org/first-year-of-life/colic/

Adaptation from Colic Calm website UK[7]

"It is not uncommon for babies to go through periods when they appear abnormally irritable, fussy or seemingly cry for no reason. However, if you suspect your baby is suffering from colic, compare your child's symptoms with the list below. Our poll of thousands of parents illustrates the frequency of nine common signs of infants with colic. Overall, 84% reported at least 5 of the signs below (see Table 1 on page 11).

Colic is often the worst pain a baby will experience. It is usually manifested as an acute abdominal pain with intense spasmodic cramping, but since colicky babies cannot describe exactly what distresses them, it is hard for parents to know the precise cause of their distress.

"Infantile colic is most common in the first few weeks to four months of an infant's life; rarely does it endure past six months of age. Paediatricians often use the "Rule of Three" to diagnose colic".

---

[7] Colic Calm, 2013-2014. *The Cause and Treatment of New-born, Infant and Baby Colic,* [Online] Available at: http://www.coliccalm.co.uk/colic.htm [Accessed 6 June 2014].

Table 1: Symptoms', Signs & Frequency of Colic

No.	Symptom / Sign	Frequency
1	Cries vigorously for long periods, despite efforts to console*	100%
2	Crying begins around the same time each day or night	77%
3	Symptoms begin after meal times	70%
4	Symptoms begin and end abruptly without warning	70%
5	Symptoms cease after a bowel movement or passing gas	62%
6	Baby spits up frequently**	46%
7	Shows signs of gas such as; abdominal bloating Or a hard distended stomach	74%
8	During episodes; baby arches back, pulls knees to chest, Clenches fists, flails arms and legs	90%
9	Baby experiences disrupted sleep patterns	83%

Notes:

1. Inconsolable crying is part of the Wessel definition of colic. Thus, all colicky infants fit these criteria.

2. The fact that relatively few reported excessive spit-up, which is quite common in babies anyway, suggests that reflux is not a factor in most cases of colic.

Recognising the Signs of Reflux

Parents are often told that they just have a fussy baby or the term "colic" may be used. Reflux is a lot different as the crying is not isolated to a specific time period and can be constant screaming and whinging night and day. I remember thinking I would swap a baby with reflux for ten babies with colic. Raven actually got diagnosed with colic on top of reflux when she was six weeks old. She would cry constantly, but for a period at night she would cry at a much higher pitch. The colic seemed to exasperate her reflux, the force of her back arching was also heightened, and trying to feed her during these hours was impossible.

Signs of Reflux

Raven displayed many traits that are common amongst babies with silent reflux (SR). Babies who repeatedly produce projectile vomit are easier to diagnose, as vomit is a more obvious visible symptom. Weight loss is also an indicator of reflux severity in some cases and it is the method used by most professionals to monitor and record the effect of reflux on the developing baby. Most babies with SR do not fall under this category as they do not lose the contents of their feed through projectile vomiting and the vital calories for weight gain are not lost. Not losing calories sometimes results in a slower diagnosis of the disease, as these babies are seen to be gaining weight; they are classed as "thriving."

Other signs include excessive crying or irritability during or after feeding or regurgitation and choking or apnoea with blue spells.

From my own experience, I found that Raven would seem extremely hungry but as soon as she would feed, within seconds, she would smack the bottle from my hand and then try to feed again. This would go on for the entire duration of her feeding time. I now know that the acid burn was obviously making drinking impossible for her.

From looking at the results of the *barium swallow test*[8] (more details in Chapter 2) we could see that the muscles in her stomach would constantly project her feed back into her oesophagus causing a counter reaction. I also remember a period of one or two months where she looked like she was drowning during feeds. This was so frightening to watch and I dreaded every single feed.

Raven would also back arch in my arms and claw at my chest and face, her arms would also fly outwards as if she had been frightened or startled.

---

[8] Mersch, John, MD, FAAP. *Barium Swallow*, Gastroesophageal Reflux (GER and GERD) in Infants and Children, P2. Available at
http://www.medicinenet.com/gerd_in_infants_and_children/article.htm [Accessed Feb 2015]

When Raven was two months old, I remember thinking she had started teething at a very young age. She had excessive drool and would eat her hands constantly. This, however, is a major symptom of reflux disease as the acid burn at the back of the throat can cause this behaviour. By means of hand chewing, the baby tries to reach the back of the throat to soothe the burn. As Raven got older she would shove her whole fist down her throat while screaming.

A baby with uncontrolled reflux will also feed voraciously. This again is their means of easing the "burn". It often results in overfeeding which in turn, will cause the reflux to worsen as there is even more milk to reflux into the oesophagus.

Sleeping patterns can be extremely poor for a lot of reflux babies. Raven would wake up numerous times at night for long periods of time. I personally find broken sleep a killer. Your day seems to pass by in a blurry haze. Concentration is lost and you feel like an emotional wreck. You feel drained with horrible brain fog. For me, sleep deprivation is my Kryptonite.

In my experience, I have found that many medical professionals are of the opinion that if a baby is thriving and gaining weight there is no cause for concern. I remember the comments about Raven during this stage and how people said she was a "fine big healthy child!" I now recoil when I hear the term "thriving."

Excessive hiccups are another significant symptom of reflux, especially wet ones. I now know when Raven is having a reflux episode because her eyes go red; she stops in her tracks and then (depending on the force) liquid can come from her nose. Another small sign of reflux is the scent of a baby's breath; it can be noticeable and sour smelling.

Many babies with reflux will have significant wind issues; this will make colic for them ten times worse. I found probiotics brilliant for this, but if your baby has intolerances to dairy choose one without. There are many different brands on the market which cater for allergies (please see chapter 7 for more information on probiotics).

Practical Ways to Manage Reflux

Keeping your baby in an upright position for 30 minutes after food can help. Elevating the cot/ Moses basket in the incline position is good. Normal baby rules seem to go out the window when dealing with a baby with GORD. If you have a good public health nurse who knows about reflux she should be able to help you with deciding what is best and safest for your baby. I had to walk around with Raven in my arms while feeding, as it was the only way she would feed. Many parents found that feeding their baby in a bouncer worked. Do whatever works best for you and your baby within reason.

Wind the baby as much as possible during and after a feed. I found that smaller feeds given more regularly made things a little easier, although this is exhausting. Some days I felt like I was constantly feeding her.

Many reflux babies do not like to be laid down on their backs; this can make the reflux unbearable as the acid can flow back up freely. Reflux babies seem to be at their best when they are being held upright and close to your chest. This is of course extremely hard to do on an on-going basis, so sling wearing is a good idea and many mothers have found them very beneficial.

I personally found a baby swing brilliant. The moving motion and being in the upright position seemed to take her mind off what was going on.

I found changing Ravens nappy before a feed helped, as I could avoid laying her down on her back afterwards.

Try to avoid overfeeding; some reflux babies will gulp their feeds to soothe the burn, and overfeeding can cause the contents of the stomach to flow more freely into the oesophagus.

Bouncing a reflux baby is not advisable either. I found the no bouncing rule hard to explain to my own parents, who a lot of the time felt I was a neurotic mother who pandered to Raven's every need.

I also avoided putting jeans or tight waist bands on her as I felt she had enough pressure inside her without adding to it.

The old cliché about bringing a crying baby out in the car does not seem to work for reflux babies. Car rides can be a nightmare; many parents have reported that they dread having to travel with their baby in the car.

I feel the position of infant baby seats can compromise a baby with reflux, as it keeps them in a bent over position. If you can, try to avoid long distance car journeys, or have someone sit in the back to distract your baby on the journey.

Using a feed thickener, such as *Carobel* (Cow and Gate), can also help babies with reflux issues, as can Comfort Feed which has a thicker consistency (See Chapter 7). These products can be beneficial for babies who vomit and for babies who have a mild form of silent reflux.

White noise can be great too, my husband would often put the hairdryer on and walk around with Raven in his arms, one mother claims they actually burnt out the hover for this very reason. The things you will do to try to help your baby are unlimited!

Black out blinds for the baby's room are excellent, we used them with soft lighting. It seemed to create a peaceful ambience and saved Raven from waking up too early during the summer months.

A portable CD player with soothing music or lullaby can help some babies to relax enough to sleep. We used to play soft music on a loop system and Raven loved it. It drove us mad, but we didn't care as it worked somewhat.

Sleep therapy can be useful for older children who have developed disrupted sleeping habits due to painful reflux. In my experience if a baby is in pain, sleep therapy will not work until the reflux is under control. A good sleep therapist should inform parents of this before beginning sessions.

There are great apps you can get for Smartphone's that play sounds. I had one of a heartbeat that Raven seemed to like; she also liked classical music and me humming in her ear as I paced the floor. Bath time is also a good way to try to calm your baby down.

Learning how to give a baby massage safely in a reclining position is also very useful and can help with colic.

I carried out a poll on my Reflux group members about the worst things that can be said to a parent with a reflux baby. From research and gathering information it seems to be the same issues for all the parents around the world. Pages 20 & 21 are supported using information provided by Reflux Infant Support Association (RISA)[9].

---

[9] Reflux Infants Support Association (RISA) Inc: http://www.reflux.org.au/ [May 15 2014]

I am Trying to Survive Reflux
Please Try To Refrain From Using The Following

1. All babies cry
2. All babies vomit
3. Is this your first
4. He's feeding off your stress
5. But she seems so happy
6. Oh my baby used to vomit all the time too
7. But he's a healthy weight?
8. Don't worry they grow out of it
9. You need to stop breast feeding/ have you tried formula
10. He's just got colic
11. She'll eat if she's hungry
12. He doesn't vomit, so it can't be reflux
13. Sleep when baby sleeps (Not helpful when baby doesn't sleep)
14. Don't let your child rule your life – They need to fit into your schedule
15. send him to me, I'll sort him out
16. Stop spoiling her
17. Your over reacting, Just relax
18. Your baby is thriving
19. He doesn't look sick
20. Screaming is good for their lungs

I'm Trying To Survive Reflux

I Really Need To Hear These Things

1. I believe you
2. It's not your fault
3. You are doing a great job – parenting a reflux baby is hard work
4. You can't spoil a reflux baby
5. This is not normal infant behaviour
6. You are not a paroniod mother: what you are feeling is normal under the circumstances
7. With the right support you will get through this
8. Let's put together a plan to help your and your baby get through this
9. It is not ok for a baby to be in pain, even if they may grow out of it in due course or never remember
10. The rules don't apply to reflux children so do what you need to do to survive; eating, sleeping and settling can be taught or modified after the pain is managed
11. A referral to _____ for support; or
12. I don't know, but I can give you a referral to someone who does

Chapter 2

A Guide to GP visits and Hospitals

When to Ask for a Paediatrician, Gastroenterologist or a Dietician.

Getting your General Practitioner (GP) or Public Health Nurse (PHN) to acknowledge that this is not the normal baby behaviour is often tough. I found that fighting hospitals and physicians were actually one of the most difficult parts of my journey. After nearly 9 months of being fobbed off we finally found a hospital and doctor that would actually listen to us.

Being prepared to go to medical appointments is absolutely vital. I would advise writing down as much as you can about how your baby is presenting, I understand that this is tough when your baby is in the throes of distress, but it will serve you well during your doctor or hospital visits.

➢ Create a diary of crying episodes and how many millilitres of formula were consumed. If you're breastfeeding, time how long your baby latched on and was feeding.

➢ Record the number of bowel movements and their consistency.

Raven had up to ten runny poos a day. They were also explosive and caused her great distress. She then developed blood in her stool, which resembled orange jelly. Raven was finally diagnosed with Cow's Milk Soy Protein Intolerance (CMSPI) .See chapter 10 for more on this condition.

➢ If possible, take video recordings with a recording device. I cannot emphasize enough the importance of this is as it shows the true nature of how things are at home for you.

I don't know how many times we ran to A&E with Raven thinking she was on her last legs, when we got there she would be like a different child, all smiles and giggles. From all the information I have gathered from my group and on my travels, this is very common in reflux babies. It appears that the new surroundings distracts them from the pain and will make you look like a complete liar, so record as much as you can.

➢ Explain everything that concerns you to your GP, including back arching, refusal to feed, vomits, constant crying etc.

If the basic reflux solutions are not working for your baby don't be afraid to ask for a referral to a paediatrician. I and others have found that most GPs are very limited in their knowledge of reflux and feel it is something a baby will simply grow out of. They can be very reluctant to prescribe medication or order further examinations.

Healthcare professionals believe that placing a baby on solids is the solution to curing reflux; on the contrary, introducing solids can make reflux a hell of a lot worse. In my experience reflux babies seem to have extremely sensitive digestive systems and will react to a lot of foods which can flare reflux.

> ➢ If you're living in Ireland and waiting lists for a paediatrician, are long in your area, I would strongly recommend going private.

It's something I regret not doing from the beginning. This can cut out so much wasted time and heartache. It will be the best money you will spend to preserve your sanity.

> ➢ Also ask for a referral to a dietician as intolerances to food go hand in hand with reflux.

Many babies with reflux also have a cow's milk intolerance. This will aggravate and flare the reflux; it is like adding fuel to a fire. No amount of medication will bring reflux under control if the suspected food is being consumed as intolerance can often be the cause of reflux in a baby.

A paediatrician may refer your baby to a paediatric gastroenterologist if your baby's symptoms require further investigation or medical procedures.

What to Bring for Hospital Admissions

We incurred four stays in two different hospitals with Raven during our reflux journey; each time made us seasoned hospital parents. Here are some suggestions of useful things to bring during your stay.

- ✓ **Baby grows/ sleeping suits, Vests, socks.**
- ✓ **Daytime wear for your child.**

I always changed Raven into these so she would know the difference between daylight and night, but it isn't essential.

- ✓ **Bring your own feeding bottles**; some babies will only tolerate their own bottles so bring plenty. Most hospitals provide a water sterilizing unit for the room, so ask for one.
- ✓ **Plenty of dummies/ pacifiers/ soothers.**

✓ **Nappies/ diapers/ cream/ wipes.**

✓ **Baby's favourite toy or music mobile** from their cot at home. Try to take in their surroundings from home to make the hospital environment as familiar as possible to them.

In my experience hospitals will not always have these to spare, so bring any activity toys you may have.

✓ **Baby car seat, stroller/Pram.**

This is extremely important as we walked many a corridor with Raven at night to try and break the cycle of her crying.

✓ For older children on solids you can **bring their preferred foods.** Please make medical staff aware of this, as they need to record all food consumed.

Most hospitals offer accommodation to parents who live long distances from the hospital, this is usually offered at a reduced price.

✓ **Call your designated hospital** to inquire about this prior to your stay as they have limited availability.

Things to Bring For Parents

Three of our hospital admissions with Raven were for observation of her pain and crying episodes. We reached the painful decision not to stay with her overnight as we wanted the medical staff to get a full picture of how things were at home for us on a constant basis.

Here are a few basic items and tips that you may find useful.

- ✓ Bring plenty of **change/coins for the parking meter**. Try sourcing information about cheap local parking places surrounding the hospital; some places offer discounts for parents who are attending the hospital. Do make yourself familiar with their parking times.
- ✓ **Wear comfortable clothing**; jeans are not a good item of clothing to sit in all day. I found that out the hard way.
- ✓ **Bring your slippers** and try not to restrict your feet. If staying overnight bring your own night clothes and toiletries.
- ✓ **Bring your laptop**; some hospitals have free Wi-Fi spots.

My husband, Lee, brought his laptop when Raven was first admitted, as he needed to finish his final year college thesis. We learned that you need to do what you can when you can as GORD is so unpredictable and time cannot easily be planned.

For example, when Raven was very young and less mobile, she was, in some respects, easier to manage. As she got bigger, more mobile and independent, it became more difficult and personal spaces during the visits got less and less.

- ✓ **A phone charger** is a must; some hospitals have a vending machine which allows you to charge your phone, which is superb.
- ✓ **Reading material** if you're lucky enough to have time and energy to read.
- ✓ **Bring plenty of money** for the canteen and vending machines. Make yourself familiar with the canteen opening and closing times.
- ✓ **Take turns with your spouse and partner** if you can; there is little point in both of you being exhausted during your stay.
- ✓ **Try to get familiar with other parents in your ward.**

Sometimes other parents can give you a more accurate picture of how your baby was in your absence. Many hospitals here in Ireland have over worked and over stretched hospital staff, sometimes things get overlooked or are not recorded properly so another set of eyes can be useful.

✓ **Try to organise child minding for other children** you may have as you don't know how long your baby may be admitted for, so be prepared and proactive.

✓ **Finally, keep your own record** of all events, feeds, crying episodes and share it with hospital staff, sometimes this can be very beneficial to both you and any medical professional involved with the care of your baby.

Diagnostic Tests for Reflux

Barium Swallow Test[10]

Definition: *"The barium Swallow Test (also called an esophagram) is a study of the oesophagus including the mouth and stomach.*

It is performed in the radiology department by a radiologist and technologist. Your baby will need to fast prior to the test. The baby will then be given a white, chalky, liquid substance to swallow from a bottle while lying down. This test is non-invasive and will cause your baby no harm or discomfort. The swallowing process is then recorded by an X-ray.

---

[10] Mersch, John, MD, FAAP. *Barium Swallow,* Gastroesophageal Reflux (GER and GERD) in Infants and Children, P2. Available at
http://www.medicinenet.com/gerd_in_infants_and_children/article.htm [Accessed Feb 2015]

The X-ray captures how the fluid flows from the mouth down the oesophagus to the stomach. This test is excellent as it shows the exact true nature of the reflux and its force. The test also checks for any abnormalities or structural defects".

PH Probe

During the test, your child is asked to swallow a long, thin tube with a probe at the tip that will stay in the oesophagus for 24 hours. The tip is positioned, usually at the lower part of the oesophagus, and measures the levels of stomach acids. It also helps determine if breathing problems are the result of reflux.

Upper GI Endoscopy

This is performed using an endoscope (a thin, flexible, lighted tube and camera) that allows the doctor to look directly inside the oesophagus, stomach, and upper part of the small intestine.

Gastric Emptying Study

Some people with GORD have slow emptying of the stomach that may be contributing to the reflux of acid. During the gastric emptying test, your child drinks milk or eats food mixed with tiny amounts of radioactive chemical. This chemical is then tracked through the gastrointestinal tract using a special camera".

Surgical Correction of Reflux – Nissen Fundoplication

Nissen Fundoplication[11]

A Nissen fundoplication is an operation used to treat gastro – oesophageal reflux.

It uses the top of the stomach to strengthen the sphincter so it is less likely to allow food, drink, or acid to travel back into the food pipe. Some babies and children have a gastrostomy, "feeding tube inserted", during the same operation.

---

[11] G.O.S., 2014. *Fundoplication - Procedures and treatments, Provided with permission from Great Ormond Street Hospital.* [Online]
Available at: http://www.gosh.nhs.uk/medical-information/procedures-and-treatments/fundoplication/

The fundoplication operation is usually carried out using keyhole surgery (laparoscopy). The surgeon uses a telescope, with a miniature video camera mounted on it, inserted through a small incision (cut) to see inside the abdomen. Carbon dioxide gas is used to inflate the abdomen to create space in which the surgeon can operate using specialised instruments that are also passed through other smaller incisions (cuts) in the abdomen.

The operation itself has two parts. Firstly, the surgeon will examine the diaphragm to check the size of the opening around the oesophagus. If it's too loose, the surgeon will tighten this. The second part of the operation involves wrapping the upper part of the stomach (fundus) around the base of the oesophagus and loosely stitching it in place. This tightens the sphincter enough to reduce reflux, but not so tight as to affect swallowing.

Although the fundoplication operation is very successful at improving a baby's gastro-oesophageal reflux disease and the symptoms associated with it, a quarter of all patients develop some long-term effects afterwards, some of which are treatable.

Changes in Feeding Pattern, Burping, Vomiting & Gas Bloat after a Nissen Fundoplication

Dumping Syndrome

This is a combination of symptoms, including nausea, retching, sweating, diarrhoea and a drop in blood sugar level. It is caused by food travelling through the stomach at a much faster rate than usual, so none of the goodness in the feed is absorbed. This can be alleviated by giving your child smaller feeds more frequently. These symptoms can take up to six weeks to settle.

Swallowing Problems: Recurrence of Reflux

In some children, reflux symptoms can come back. This is because the fundoplication is failing (coming undone). Your surgeon may recommend that the operation is performed again or that alternative methods of managing reflux should be investigated"

Parents Experience

"My son was born in September 2012 with a congenital disorder called Oesophageal Atresia. His oesophagus was not connected so he could not eat, drink or swallow. It's very rare in Ireland and

33

is diagnosed at the 20 week scan. He spent 6 months in a Children's Hospital in Ireland, where they could not fix him so we went to Poland (we're Irish, but the surgeon was there) with the Treatment Abroad scheme.

However, we still needed to do some fund raising in order to cover our daily living expenses and bills. We spent 3 months there where they did the Foker procedure (Developed by John Foker, MD, a Paediatric surgeon from the University of Minnesota) to fix him (major surgery). The Foker process [12] *is a technique to stimulate the upper and lower ends of the oesophagus to grow so they could be joined together. It is only available in Boston's Children's Hospital, USA and Gdansk Hospital, Poland.*

The USA was not an option for us, but we were referred to Poland by the Boston Children's Hospital. After he was fixed he

---

[12] Boston Children's Hospital, Esophageal Atresia in Children. Reviewed by Russell W. Jennings, MD © Children's Hospital Boston; posted in 201. [Accessed Feb 2015] Available online at:

http://www.childrenshospital.org/conditions-and-treatments/conditions/esophageal-atresia.

had Pyloric Stenosis and chronic Reflux. It was so bad he had to have a Nissen Fundoplication which resolved his reflux. However, he will be on Losec (10mg currently) for life. He was also peg tube for just under 2 years. He got his peg out last month. He is a miracle baby as he loves food (though still only on purees) and has caught up developmentally. He requires dilations when his oesophagus strictures.

We go to Poland for these. Our son's long term outcome is positive. In fact, the Foker process most often results in an oesophagus that's indistinguishable from one that has developed normally. Our goal was 'short term pain for long term gain'. Although it's been a nightmare of a journey, ours can have a happy ending. He is a very happy little boy and will not remember all the surgery he has been through. In fact, he loves nothing more than to play with his 4 year old sister."

Chapter 3

Tube Feeding

The following information has been kindly provided by

Suzanne Evans Morris, Ph.D.

[13] *"Children who receive all or part of their nourishment through a tube create special challenges for therapists and parents. There is a tendency for others to view the tube as an enemy of progress as something to be gotten rid of. Children are often referred to a therapist with the specific request to get the child off the tube and onto oral feedings as rapidly as possible. When the transition to oral feeding is not made rapidly, everyone feels like a failure. With many children, the emphasis has been placed on the feeding process, rather than on the development of skills that could support feeding. This is rather like putting the cart before the*

---

[13] Suzanne Evans Morris, Ph.D, Children with Feeding Tubes, [online] [Accessed Mar 2015] available at http://www.new-vis.com/fym/papers/p-feed12.htm

36

horse. Let us review the special questions, issues, and problems that are presented when a child has a severe feeding problem that requires tube feeding.

Why are Feeding Tubes Recommended?

Tube feedings can be initiated for a wide variety of reasons. Premature infants under the gestational age of 33 weeks or 3 pounds have not reached the stage of development where strong sucking and swallowing patterns can support oral feedings. Some children have such severe respiratory or cardiac problems that they do not have the energy to suck and swallow. Because the respiratory system and the feeding system use the same passageway in the upper portion of the pharynx, difficulties with swallowing or breathing can cause a child to aspirate, or draw food or liquid into the lungs rather than into the esophagus. Other children may lack the neurological coordination required to organize the collection and movement of food in the mouth, and to propel it to the back of the tongue and the pharynx for swallowing. Sucking and swallowing may be very slow or extremely uncoordinated, and the child might be unable to take in enough calories before becoming exhausted. Still other children experience severe gastrointestinal difficulties that cause food to be refluxed and vomited. Surgical procedures to prevent reflux may increase the discomfort of swallowing and result in a reduced desire to eat.

What Characteristics are seen in Children who are Tube-Fed?

Children who are tube-fed have many characteristics in common with other children with feeding problems. Other characteristics appear to be unique to the child with a severe feeding disorder. The severity or special combination of these characteristics prevents the infant from achieving many of the developmental feeding abilities that would be seen normally at 1-2 months of age. Two of more of the following physical and sensory behaviours have been observed consistently in infants under 18 months who have been placed on tube-feedings:

- ✓ *__Hyperextension__ of the neck, accompanied by scapular adduction and shoulder girdle elevation is seen as the primary movement characteristic of many of these infants. These tone and movement patterns strongly influence the infant's feeding and respiratory abilities.*

38

✓ **Respiratory difficulties** *are observed with high frequency. These generally reflect in the coordination of sucking and swallowing patterns with breathing. Respiratory control problems contribute to fearfulness and caution as a general approach to new or unsuccessful experiences. Respiratory problems may become exaggerated when the child produces excessive mucous that collects in the pharyngeal airway. Infants with primary respiratory dysfunction related to prematurity or cardiac disorders are often unable to coordinate a suck-swallow-breathe pattern. Their energy is directed toward the breathing portion of this triad. The baby temporarily may have an absent swallow reflex, or may refuse to take the nipple when it is offered.*

✓ **Dysfunctional and disorganized sucking patterns** *are characteristic of the majority of tube-fed infants with prematurity or neurological dysfunction. A clear sucking rhythm is often lacking. Movements may be further disorganized when touch or pressure is applied to the tongue with a nipple or spoon. The disorganized infant may use a rapid, non-nutritive suck with the bottle, or may forget to pause for breathing in the suck-swallow-breathe cycle.*

✓ ***Swallowing disorders*** *preclude the development of successful oral feeding. The infant may have difficulty using the tongue and lips to organize the bolus of food or liquid in the oral cavity and project it backward for the swallow. Small amounts of food may drip over the back of the tongue without causing a swallowing reflex to be elicited. When the swallowing reflex fails to occur, the airway is open and unprotected, and the upper end of esophagus does not open to allow the passage of food. Aspiration of the food into the lungs is the natural consequence. Some children have a swallowing reflex that is delayed. Instead of the pattern triggering from the backward movement of the tongue and the stimulation of the anterior pillars of fauces, the reflex will be elicited after food or liquid has collected in the valleculae or pyriform sinuses. Although the swallow occurs, a portion of the bolus may be aspirated before or after the swallow.*

✓ ***Hypersensitive responses to oral stimulation*** *occur frequently when the infant has been deprived of positive sensory input to the mouth. When sensory input is provided, it may be experienced as very strong and uncomfortable. Since many children require invasive procedures such as suctioning and tube-insertion, a belief that the mouth is an unpleasant place can* *develop. The infant avoids using the mouth to explore and learn because it is uncomfortable. He becomes wary and watchful of anyone who approaches his mouth, assuming that the sensory input will be intensely uncomfortable*

✓ ***Sensory defensive responses*** *to facial and oral stimulation occur as a primary difficulty in some children. Defensive responses are strongly negative, and throw the child immediately into a fight-or-flight reaction. The child's basic perception is one of danger, and the sensory stimulus is often perceived as an attack. Sensory defensiveness may occur as a response to touch, movement, smell, taste, and texture in food.*

✓ ***Gastroesophageal reflux*** *occurs when the muscles at the lower end of the esophagus fail to contract enough to prevent reflux or backwash of stomach contents into the esophagus and pharynx. Reflux often results in vomiting. Reflux is unpleasant for the child and caregivers. Constant acid irritation of the esophagus can reduce the infant's desire to take food by mouth because of the discomfort.*

✓ *Delayed gastric emptying* is observed when food remains in the stomach and is not efficiently emptied into the small intestine. This condition contributes to gastroesophageal reflux and to a reduction in appetite. When the stomach contains a substantial amount of food from the last meal, children aren't hungry when the next meal is offered.

✓ *Gagging, retching, and nausea* occur when the gastrointestinal system is under severe stress. These symptoms are most common as a side-effect of medication, or gastrointestinal surgery. Children whose reflux has been stopped with a fundoplication may begin to retch during or between tube feedings. This unproductive heaving and gagging is extremely distressing to the child and family, and strongly reduces the desire to eat. When gastric emptying is delayed, a pyloroplasty may be added to the fundoplication, creating an open valve at the bottom of the stomach to enhance gastric emptying. Some children experience rapid dumping of stomach contents into the intestines following this procedure. Sudden changes in blood sugar and autonomic nervous system symptoms such as sweating, pallor, and nausea may accompany tube feedings.

✓ *Eating aversion is the result of a complex interplay of sensorimotor, gastrointestinal, and environmental responses. It is a term used to describe children who simply do not want to eat. It is typically perceived as a behavioural issue, with the child confronting adults with a strong refusal to accept enough food to be adequately nourished. The term infantile anorexia is occasionally used to describe these children. However, a large number of these children have subtle sensorimotor and gastrointestinal characteristics that make eating uncomfortable. These children may choose a non-eating behaviour to reduce or prevent discomfort. This choice may become strong and unbending when the child experiences pressure from others to eat.*

✓ *Failure-to-thrive is the end result of physical, sensory, metabolic, or environmental eating difficulties. The child does not gain grow adequately with oral feeding. Tube feedings may be initiated as a temporary measure to increase the child's nutritional status and improve growth.*

What Types of Feeding Tubes Are Recommended for Children?

Tubes can be divided into two general categories: those that are inserted through the oral-pharyngeal area (i.e. nasogastric tubes, orogastric tubes), and those that are not (i.e. gastrostomy tubes, jeujenostomy tubes). This is an important distinction therapeutically. The insertion and presence of a tube in the nose, mouth, or pharynx may actually compete with goals of an oral-motor treatment program. Since one of the goals in the program is to develop a sense of pleasure and enjoyment with use of the mouth, this will become more difficult if tubes must constantly be inserted or remain in the naso-pharyngeal area.

It is also uncomfortable for some children to actively suck and swallow with the tube in place. Added breathing difficulties can arise when one small nostril of an infant is occluded by the tube. Although the nasogastric tube is usually the first tube a child receives, it has many disadvantages when used as a long-term procedure.

If the child is a candidate for surgical procedures, the insertion of a gastrostomy tube can enable nourishment to be supplied in a way that does not conflict with oral-motor treatment goals. The area of invasion for the tube is separated from the oral-pharyngeal area. It becomes much easier for the child to discover the pleasurable aspects of the mouth. Because there is no longer a tube taped across the face, the child looks less ill, and the parents are subjected to fewer stares and questions.

There are disadvantages to the gastrostomy tube that must be considered. Surgery is risky for some children, even when it is done without general anaesthesia (i.e. PEG procedure). Some children develop a mild irritation and leakage around the tube site. This can be uncomfortable for the child and of concern to the parents. A gastrostomy procedure can increase the risk of gastroesophageal reflux or make an existing reflux disorder more severe. When reflux is present or suspected, more extensive surgery is usually combined with the insertion of a gastrostomy tube. The most common procedure, the Nissen fundoplication, creates a wrap of stomach tissue around the lower esophageal sphincter to prevent the refluxing of stomach contents into esophagus. When the gastroesophageal reflux is a symptom of a more extensive disorder of the gastrointestinal system, severe side effects can result.

Many children with neurological dysfunction show poor motility of the entire system. The stomach empties too slowly, and movement of digested food through the intestines may be slow or reduced. The fundoplication may contribute to gagging, retching, gas bloat, nausea,

45

and other major discomforts that reduce the child's interest in taking food orally.

If reflux is severe, a tube may be inserted directly into the jejunum at the top of the small intestines, bypassing the stomach. This eliminates the risk of refluxing food from the stomach. Stomach acids and other secretions may, however, still be refluxed.

Some children are unable to absorb adequate nutrients through the intestinal walls because of shortening of the intestinal tract or lack of intestinal motility. Nutrients can be given through a central line that goes directly into the blood stream. This is referred to as hyperalimentation or TPN (total parenteral nutrition).

Does Tube Feedings Ever Reduce the Child's Ability or Desire to Eat Orally?

When tube feedings are initiated immediately after birth, the infant lacks the opportunity to build associations between positive sensations in the mouth and the reduction of hunger, or the social interaction with another person that surrounds a meal. If oral feedings become possible at a later time, the prime associations and motivations to take food by mouth will be missing. The child may see no relationship between learning to handle food in the mouth and the satisfying inner feelings that come after a good meal. This can become a greater barrier to the establishment of oral feedings than the original sensorimotor problem.

Tube feedings may initiate or increase gastroesophageal reflux. When reflux occurs regularly, esophageal irritation and pain can result. As this becomes associated with mealtimes, the young child may connect eating with being uncomfortable. This reduces the desire to taste food and eat by mouth.

When total tube feedings are initiated in a child who has been taking food orally, the mouth may go through many changes. The stimulation provided by touch to the mouth, feeding utensils (i.e. nipples, spoons, cups), and food often disappears from the child's sensory experience. Small sucking and swallowing movements that may have been present, but inadequate to support nutrition, are no longer stimulated and practiced. Over time, they appear to be forgotten and do not occur when a nipple or food is placed in the mouth. Negative and invasive stimulation to the face and mouth continues or increases as suctioning, intubation, tube insertion, and other life-enhancing procedures are carried out.

Gradually the mouth becomes unfamiliar with touch, taste, texture, and other stimuli that had pleasurable associations.

The face and mouth can become physically hypersensitive to touch and taste when a child has not experienced this type of input for a long time. It is as if the nervous system increases its sensitivity to search for input that has been withdrawn with the addition of tube feedings. When sensory input is provided, it is perceived as invasive, uncomfortable, sudden, and intense. The infant dislikes the way things feel and taste in he mouth. If there are problems with physical coordination, the baby may be unable to put fingers, fists, and toys in the mouth. He is unable to participate in the exploration that is the primary path to learning in the infant and young child. Because most of the sensory input that is given is provided by another person, the infant becomes cautious about allowing anyone near the mouth.

Much of the sensory input that is provided by others is uncomfortable and unpleasant. Suctioning and insertion of a nasogastric or orogastric tube occurs frequently for many medically-at-risk infants. With each invasion of the oral space, the child strengthens a belief that sensations in the mouth are dangerous and unpleasant. An unending circle begins as the infant erects barriers against anyone who would provide oral stimulation or offer food.

How Can Parents Support the Child's Desire and Ability to Eat Orally?

Children who receive tube-feedings should have the opportunity to develop comfortable and safe oral-motor skills through a specialized therapy program. However, there are many things that parents can do to support the child's ability to return to some oral feeding in the future.

Children's tube-feeding mealtimes contribute to their associations with food and being fed. When mealtimes are relaxed, comfortable, and interactive, the child learns that eating can be pleasurable. An infant can be cradled in the parent's arms for a tube-feeding and receive the same interactive benefits with a caring feeder as a bottle-fed infant. Older infants and toddlers can be tube-fed during a family meal or fed in a special chair or location associated with eating.

If gastrointestinal discomfort is present during tube-feedings, special attention can be given to reducing stress associated with mealtimes. Children and their parents often anticipate retching or vomiting which adds to the overall stress level and physical discomfort. The anticipatory stress often serves as a trigger that increases both the frequency and severity of the reflux. Activities that calm and relax the child can be used to prepare the child for the meal. Music can support physical and mental relaxation. Parents can learn to recognize the child's first signals of discomfort. The flow of formula can be stopped before the child becomes distressed. Multiple pauses during the meal can reduce the triggers that initiate episodes of severe reflux, vomiting, or retching.

Loving, interactive sensory input can be provided to the child's face and mouth during play and daily care activities. Comforting touch, patting or stroking while signing or making funny sounds together can build positive associations with orofacial input. This can prevent hypersensitivity and negative associations from developing.

If the child does not experience reflux or other gastrointestinal discomfort during the meal, oral stimulation can be provided during tube feedings. This can include sucking on a pacifier, stroking the lips, playing with mouth toys or other positive input. This is used to help the child maintain or develop oral-motor skills that can be used for oral feeding at a later point".

Mother Voices & Experience

Jennifer Green

In my own experience tube feeding can also lead to further issues such as oral aversions, causing a child to regress with what little skills they already had.

In severe cases even when a child does oral feed they can lose most of the feed through vomiting and can require slow tube feeding to allow the body to absorb the feed without triggering the reflux.

Fundoplication surgery these days is usually considered when a child has a severe reflux that they don't feel they will grow out of or if they have other co-morbidities that complicate their reflux, such as aspiration. The risk to the lungs from having acid and milk in them is very high and can cause a child to be very poorly with pneumonia. In these cases fundoplication surgery can work very well.

Playing around with the speed in which tube feeds are given can often help if a child is getting discomfort. Often it is being given too fast for the tummy to deal with. Especially if you think about when you drink, you would take breaks and drink slowly; often slowing down the feed will help.

Jack's Story

My eldest son Jack was born in March 2002 when I was still very naive about motherhood and hadn't even heard of reflux. From his very first week we had sick, we were told by the health visitor that this was normal and all babies were sick after feeding. Even hours after a feed they told me. When he was 5 weeks old, he was sick, but seemed to choke on it, his lips went blue and we rushed to the hospital. This is the first time that someone mentioned reflux; they sent us home with infant Gaviscon and thickener which these days aren't supposed to be given together. (They both thicken so shouldn't be used together) and told us that he was thriving and would be ok. They also said he would grow out of it by the time he was 6 months old.

These medications made little difference to our lives, Jack was miserable and we were miserable and our paediatrician at the time kept telling me that he was fine as he was gaining weight and that reflux was a social problem that affected me more than him.

We spent the day holding him upright and hoping he would settle. The doctors would tell my health visitor that I was anxious, I was young, and that I needed support. We felt like we didn't fit anywhere, we couldn't go to baby gym because he would vomit, or scream the whole time. We had started taking cot sheets in the nappy bag instead of muslins as they *were much bigger to clean up his vomit. We had cut his shirt off several times as I just couldn't bring myself to unbutton it.*

As luck would have it at 7 months our doctor left on maternity leave and we got our amazing consultant that we still have today.

I explained to her that we had been made to feel that we couldn't cope with our own child because people kept saying its normal. She checked him over and found a heart murmur that turned out to be innocent but the other doctor hadn't said anything anytime she had seen him.

She then referred jack to a bigger teaching hospital where they would do some tests to see how bad his reflux was and she also gave us ranitidine to try in the meantime. Jack went into the hospital where he had a pH. Study and an endoscopy, which showed that he, had quite significant reflux that wasn't being controlled; they recommended that we start omeprazole and also a low dose of erythromycin. Omeprazole helps with the acid and erythromycin to help speed up the stomach emptying to try and stop the vomiting.

We slowly over time increased this dose to what was considered maximum and he would still reflux. As he was getting older we could see that he was eating less and less and would refuse food. He would only eat yogurt and scrambled eggs at one point as I think he found that these hurt him less. Obviously with this drop his previous good weights had begun to falter, this and the fact that he was still refluxing past the age of two made them repeat the reflux tests to see if there had been any improvements.

After the test it showed the start of irritation to his oesophagus (esophagitis) and also showed that his reflux hadn't got any better but in fact showed it was worse than it had 18 months previously.

After a lot of discussion with the surgeons it was decided that the best way forward was to have a Nissans fundoplication surgery done and also a gastrostomy feeding tube placed at the same time.

This was all new to us. Our baby boy needing an operation, we hadn't even thought about the feeding tube, I was just so upset at the thought of him having a scar.

I spoke to other parents before the operation to see what they had been through, read up about what the operation did and how to care for a PEG feeding tube. I couldn't even say gastrostomy on the day of his surgery; I called it gastronomy for weeks.

Jack had the surgery in September 2004 and for us the surgery was life changing. Honestly Jack is now 13 years old and he hasn't refluxed since, sadly because of his oral aversions from being sick and the fact that we didn't get any sensory input back then means that he still doesn't eat

54

very well now and is still fed via a gastrostomy tube. He is eating orally now and he will even drink a few of the supplement drinks, but the rest we put down the tube. We, however live in hope that he will eventually be able to get off the feeding tube.

Looking back, I can't believe that I would be ever afraid of the feeding tube. It has been life changing. It took the pressure off mealtimes, stopped us being stressed about if he had had enough to eat or drink that day.

It stopped hospital admissions for bugs because we could keep him hydrated at home; we could always get medication in when other families were struggling because it didn't taste nice.

It just helped, a lot.

We did try for a year to tube wean and actually stopped all feeds but jack stopped growing completely and soon had faltering growth again so we had to put him back on full feeds.

It is rare that children with reflux don't grow out of it by Jack's age and just recently Jack and my other two children have been diagnosed with a genetic condition called Ehlers Danlos syndrome, which can cause the sphincter muscle at the top of the stomach to stay floppy which can attribute to reflux. Jack also has ADHD and anxiety; although these aren't related to reflux they could be part of the reason for him not eating. It finally gave us an answer as to why us.

This was our legacy from reflux. I believe it was from being pushed away from help for so long and then not getting input from services. In 2002 it was rare for a child to need surgery who didn't have a neurological condition. These children are already known to services which is why we slipped through the net.

Jack's Story Continued: Story about Grieving for the Life you Wanted

I made peace with my life a long time ago now, but it took a long time. I'm writing this so other parents who have children with additional needs don't feel like it's something to be ashamed of.

Grieving seems an odd thing for a person to do when they have a family and no one has died and I felt exactly the same.

I felt that I should be grateful that I had my baby when so many others left the hospital empty handed or couldn't even get a baby to start with.

I had my husband and my house and a very, very good supportive family around me.

Then, the butt's start

I didn't have the healthiest child that I had dreamed I would get,

I feel that I missed my child's first year because instead of being a mum, I was a nurse.

I was making sure that my children got the right amount of medication and that food didn't contain dairy for my daughter.

I felt like I didn't fit in at the baby clinic. I was the lady with the poorly baby, the one with the tube, or the one who is sick all the time.

We missed birthdays and family parties due to being sat in a hospital.

I spent a year with my eldest being made think that I couldn't cope with my own child, that reflux was a social problem that affected me more than him, that I was an anxious mum, a young mum, being made feel useless and that I had to fight to get listened to and get Jack treated.

This wouldn't happen for other illnesses, but people don't understand the impact that reflux can have on a child, a family, a life. This is the reason I was made to feel the way, with comments like all babies are sick. "Oh yes, my son has reflux too, he was sick once a week and sleeps all night" people that say, "oh I was up all night", but actually they had been up twice in two minutes and you had been up 4 times for an hour stripping beds and washing everything.

With my daughter, I find it hard to remember what age she was when she first crawled or her first tooth, yet I can tell you how many calories per ml her feed was and how many ml an hour she was on.

I didn't get the baby moon that everyone else gets as I was fighting to keep my baby out of hospital and then fighting to keep a smile on my face, to make sure the health visitor didn't think I was anxious or struggling. Making sure everyone thought life was good and that I was fine.

It took years and then only when I saw it in other parents to realise that I was grieving for my baby moon, for the life I thought I was getting, for the months and years that I missed out on being mum and not mum, nurse, dietician.

I felt powerless, out of control, lost, alone, lonely, but it is a feeling that passes and I think it passes because I accepted that actually it is OK to grieve and then move on, we all have that right. It shouldn't have to be a taboo to be upset.

Chapter 4

Tongue Tie and Breast Feeding

Information kindly provided by Carmen Fernando[14]

Tongue Tie

"Tongue Tie – also known as 'Ankyloglossia' or 'anchored tongue' – is a common but often overlooked condition. Tongue tie can be defined as a structural abnormality of the lingual frenum (a small fold of mucous membrane extending from the floor of the mouth to the midline of the underside of the tongue).

When the frenum is normal, it is elastic and does not interfere with the movements of the tongue in sucking, eating, clearing food off the teeth in preparation for swallowing and, of course, in speech.

---

[14] Web Development © 2007 Invisible Ink, 2007. *Tounge-Tie: From Confusion To Clarity.* [Online] Available at: http://www.tonguetie.net/index.php?option=com_frontpage&Itemid=1 [Accessed 18 May 2014].

When the tongue is short, thick, tight or broad it has an adverse effect on oro-muscular function, feeding and speech. It can also cause problems when it extends from the margin of the tongue and across the floor of the mouth to finish at the base of the teeth.

Appearance

Not all tongue ties look alike, adding to the difficulty of spotting them. They can be thin and membranous, thick and white, short, long or wide, extending from the margin of the tongue all the way to the lower front teeth, or so short and tight that they make a web connecting the tongue to the floor of the mouth. When they extend to the margin of the tongue, a heart-shaped look at the front of the tongue and no tongue tip can be seen. When a tongue tie extends across the floor of pain will be felt when the tongue is elevated. They can cause separation or inward tilting of the incisors. A baby with a tongue tie will look different from an older child with the same condition.

Intervention

Up to the year 1940, tongue ties were routinely cut to help feeding. When this changed because of a fear of excessive/unnecessary surgery and a reduction in the practice of breastfeeding, the belief that tongue tie was not a "real" medical problem but an idea held by over-zealous parents became widespread.

Early intervention is ideal since it avoids habit formation and the negative effects of failure, whether it is due to messy or slow eating, abnormal looking teeth or speech problems. When there are no strong habits to eradicate there is a better chance of success in correcting the difficulties that poor tongue mobility has caused.

Once a tongue tie has been diagnosed, the primary need is to correct the structural anomaly causing the problem. After the structural problem has been successfully corrected, it is reasonable to expect to improve function, and to treat secondary problems successfully. The type of treatment that is most appropriate depends on the problems that have been experienced.

A lactation consultant can help with correcting poor sucking which will improve breastfeeding. A speech-language pathologist will help with speech and language problems. A dentist or orthodontist can help with problems of crooked or decayed teeth and infected gums[15].

Breast Feeding

The impact of a significant tongue tie on the ability of a baby to be breastfed is very often severe. As a consequence, many mothers who plan to breastfeed their babies are compelled to wean them to the bottle much earlier than expected.

It is not always possible to predict which tongue ties will inhibit breastfeeding, as characteristics of the mother's breasts also have an effect on factors such as milk transfer. The length of the frenum (or the apparent severity of the tongue tie) has no bearing on whether the baby will be able to breastfeed efficiently.

---

[15] Weidman Sterling, Evelina, Best-Boss, Angie, Your Child's Teeth: A Complete Guide for Parents . [Online] Available at https://books.google.ie/books?isbn=142141063X - 2013 - Health & Fitness. [Accessed Feb 2015]

The Process of Breast Feeding

Milk develops in the mother's breast after the birth of her baby, but the supply is replenished and increased only by the vigorous sucking that empties the breast. If the baby cannot suck correctly, the milk supply is not renewed and it is very likely that it will eventually fail.

The infant needs to open the mouth widely enough (gaping) to allow the tongue to protrude forward, past the gum ridge, and then it must take a big mouthful of the breast. This ensures that the milk sinuses are massaged by movements of the baby's tongue and by pressure from the lower alveolar ridge causing the release of milk which is ejected through the nipple.

The tongue protruding over the gum ridge protects the nipple from being squashed painfully and even damaged by being caught repeatedly between the upper and lower gums.

Peristaltic movement of the tongue, (rippling, from the front of the tongue to the back), strokes the breast, draws out and maintains the flow of milk.

These movements of the tongue also stimulate the nipple to elongate, so that it is pointing down the baby's throat, and directing milk towards the esophagus. Most babies can empty a breast in 10 to 15 minutes with efficient sucking.

When there is a surge in the production of milk, which flows more strongly for a while, it is called 'let-down'.

The Tongue-Tied Baby

When a tongue tie is causing problems with breastfeeding, the baby often does not open his mouth widely, thus not latching on to the breast at the correct angle. Instead, he may latch onto the nipple, and 'gum' or chew it, causing severe pain and eventually, nipple damage. There can be cracking, distortion, blanching or bleeding from the nipple, sometimes followed by infection or mastitis.

The tongue tied baby also will be unable to protrude the tongue horizontally past the gum ridge or lips, because of tension on the short or tight frenum in this posture. The mother's nipple is therefore not protected from injury.

Peristaltic movement may not occur at all, it may occur only on one side of the tongue, or it may even occur irregularly. In some cases it may even change to a reverse peristalsis, with the ripple going from the back of the tongue to the front.

The nipple does not elongate, and milk may not be directed correctly for swallowing, making the baby prone to aspiration of fluids, infections, coughing, gagging, choking, or vomiting.

Since the latch is not correctly positioned, the sinuses where milk is stored are not stimulated to release milk.

The tongue-tied baby may be found to be unable to make a good seal around the breast with his lips so that milk is seen to dribble from the mouth while sucking. This is sometimes due to the presence of a maxillary frenum - a prolonged or tight frenum between the upper lip and the upper gum which limits the flexibility or mobility of the upper lip - which can be present together with a tongue tie.

Noisy sucking or noisy snap-back sucking is often reported, where the frenum stretches as far as it can go to compress the nipple, and then snaps back like a stretched rubber band being released. This can occur with both breast and bottle feeding.

Since latch is often not correctly positioned, the mother suffers intense pain when the baby seizes the nipple or chews on it, or even when he slides off the nipple, being unable to maintain a hold on the breast. In some cases the pain is severe enough to make mothers dread breastfeeding.

Maternal nipple pain is reported to preclude an adequate milk ejection reflex, and the presence of all or even some of the above problems can interfere with the acquisition of milk. The unsatisfied infant, tired out with sucking, but comfortable in his mother's arms will often fall asleep on the breast, only to waken still hungry and needing further feeding.

Some mothers have reported feeding their baby 2 hourly, day and night; others describe a feed that might last 2 hours. Pain from such continuous feeding can be so severe that mothers reported hoping their babies would continue sleeping.

These problems can persist in spite of help and support from professionals. Doctors are often unable to help these mothers, who are told that the nipples will toughen up, or even to take painkillers prior to feeding. Unfortunately the pain will only abate if the structural problem is corrected.

The infant can experience as much discomfort as the mother: hunger, malnourishments, swallowing of wind, sleep disturbances, vomiting, and reflux can be present, causing incessant crying and inability to settle.

Breastfeeding in these circumstances will be anything but pleasurable or satisfying and will cause disappointment, sadness and guilt for the mother. Poor weight gain or failure to thrive may prompt termination of breastfeeding and early weaning to the bottle.

Some infants will continue to have problems on the bottle, such as dribbling, swallowing of air and vomiting. Many will also have difficulty coping with purees and solids when these are introduced.

Conclusion

It is still possible to find items in the literature on Ankyloglossia which state that tongue tie does not inhibit breastfeeding or cause other significant problems. However, there is also a growing body of evidence - both anecdotal and scientific - from studies and trials which indicates that tongue tie does affect breastfeeding strongly enough to interrupt it.

Parents Views

"My baby had tongue tie but was bottle fed. Got it snipped 5 weeks ago-much better feeder".

"Tongue-tie correction at 8 weeks but had abandoned breast-feeding at that point. It made no difference to latch or colic & reflux".

"Had it snipped at 3 weeks, huge improvement and was able to continue breastfeeding as a result".

"I found it improved things greatly for us".

"My little girl has grade 4/3 tongue tie but didn't need to be snipped".

Chapter 5

Feeding & Baby Formula

I strongly believe that breastfeeding is a better option for babies in general, it is certainly best for babies with reflux as it is easier for them to digest and has all the natural nutrients required to maintain a healthy child. However, breastfeeding was not an option for me as Raven had so many intolerances and her reflux was so severe.

I was exhausted and had zero time to prepare special meals for myself that were free from dairy and soy. I existed on coffee, tea, soft drinks and snacks, anything I could eat quickly and easily. I would have totally believed that my milk was making her sick if I continued, more guilt, more doubt, on top of everything. I hadn't the mental strength to handle all that, so we decided that formula feeding was best for us.

If you are struggling with breastfeeding your baby, please contact you're nearest certified lactation consultant; a list of specialists can be found on http://www.alcireland.ie/. Try and exhaust all areas before deciding to formula feed your baby, but please go easy on yourself, I regret not feeding Raven myself but at the time it was the best thing for both of us.

There are so many different baby formulas on the market designed to help babies with reflux. I can't remember how many different formulas Raven was on before we got the right balance.

This chapter will give brief information about suitable baby formulas and provides random tried and tested reviews from parents in the SRI group.

Hipp Organic Combiotic Follow On from 6 Months Onwards (UK)

This formula is specially formulated using organic milk. It is gentle and contains probiotic oligosaccharides which support the growth of healthy bacteria in your baby's tummy. It also contains naturally occurring Omega 3 (alpha linolenic acid) which is important for healthy brain and nervous system development (Suitable only from six months).

This baby formula was well tolerated amongst babies who could have dairy. This formula contains no synthetic forms of DHA (docosahexaenoic acid) or ARA (arachidonic acid)

Parent's Review

"We found *this formula brilliant for our baby and she loved the taste luckily she has no intolerances so it was fine for us".*

SMA Advanced Gold System

This range encompasses a range of scientifically developed formulas to help meet the nutritional needs of babies and young children. Every product has a tailored nutrient profile for each stage of growth and development.

SMA, WySoy Soya Infant Milk from Birth Onwards

This nutritionally complete soya infant formula is suitable for babies and young children who are intolerant to cow's milk, when they are not being breastfed. It can be used as the sole source of nutrition in the early months and used in place of the milk part of a mixed diet as your baby gets older. Here is a manufacturers' list of some of the special features of this formula:

71

- When baby needs a milk free diet.
- Part of the Advanced Gold System.
- Nutritionally complete cow's milk free formula.
- Omega 3 & 6 LCPs long chain polyunsaturates.
- Specially tailored use as a drink or in recipes.
- Vegetarian Society approved.
- Suitable for Halal.

SMA Nutrition Range

This range contains many products to help suit babies' feeding needs.

Allergy Information: Contains: Soya\Soybeans

Parent's Review

"My little boy wouldn't drink much breast milk or Aptamil Formula. The doctor thought he just had a latching problem which would sort itself out. So we were advised to force-feed him, which would leave him screaming when doing so. We were at the hospital, GP or health nurse all the time as he was not gaining enough weight, etc. I changed him onto SMA WySoy as I

believed he was drinking enough but wasn't able to digest the nutrients in normal formula properly. He is a completely different baby now. He looks for his bottles, which is shocking for me to see. He is gaining weight as he should be. The doctor wasn't happy with my decision to change him to WySoy he told me to wean him onto normal SMA. Never again! He really screamed all day! He was in so much pain and this was only a scoop in his normal bottle. I swear by SMA WySoy and I don't intend to change again".

Aptamil & Cow & Gate, Comfort Formula

The comfort formula is designed for the dietary management of colic and constipation. These ranges of foods are for special medical purposes. These are available from birth upwards.

- Designed for the dietary management of colic and constipation following consultation with your healthcare professional
- Aptamil Comfort is suitable from birth.
- Nutritionally complete, you can be confident that your little one is getting everything they need.

73

- Partially hydrolysed proteins and a special fat blend are gentle on baby's digestive system
- Prebiotics oligosaccharides help to soften stools.
- Also contains nucleotides and long chain polyunsaturated fatty acids (LCPs)

Aptamil *Comfort* is nutritionally tailored with a unique blend of GOS/FOS prebiotics helping to soften stools. It also contains nucleotides and antioxidants, and has milk proteins which have been partially broken down (partially hydrolysed) to make them much gentler on your baby's digestive system. Aptamil *Comfort* also contains long chain polyunsaturated fatty acids (LCPs) from the omega-3 and omega-6 groups, which means that bottle-fed babies suffering from colic and constipation can get the benefits of LCPs up to the age of one year.

Due to *Aptamil Comfort* being slightly thicker than other milks, you may find that a variable flow teat or a single whole teat with a medium or fast flow is better when feeding your baby.

We tried this formula before Raven had been diagnosed with cow's milk soy protein intolerance and although she loved the taste and we did find the consistency thicker, it was not suitable for Raven.

Parent's Review

"Harry was on Aptamil Comfort, it was great to keep him regular but he still had spit up. He has no allergies, his reflux I think is caused by low muscle tone, hypertonia. His poos were a bit free at the start, but that's only with the change from normal Aptamil, from 6 months he was on Hipp Organic a lovely formula for babies with no allergies. I also have him on Dr Udos[16], and he was on Losec 10 mg till 12 months! Med free now and reflux gone! Still gets the odd hiccups, a bit of gripe water helps!"

Aptamil, Pepti 1

Aptamil *Pepti 1* is a food for special medical purposes for the dietary management of cow's milk protein allergy (CMPI). The cow's milk protein in *Aptamil Pepti 1* has been hydrolysed or broken down into

---

[16] Udo Erasmus, Fats That Heal, Fats That Kill, Published December 1st 1998 by Alive Books (first published January 1st 1993) Product referred to is UDO'S CHOICE Infant's Blend, GUT MICROFLORA PREPARATION, Information Available at: http://.udoschoice.co.uk/products

smaller 'pieces' which makes it easier to tolerate and digest for babies with cow's milk protein allergy. *Aptamil Pepti 1* is a nutritionally complete formula, suitable from birth, and can also be used to replace cow's milk in drinks and cooked dishes during and after weaning.

Parent's Review

"Our Baby was on Pepti 1 for 2 months for CMPI, it smells horrible and our baby was reluctant to take it. Did work for the first while, but then as it turned out she's lactose intolerant and it contains lactose."

"We changed after visit to A&E at 6 weeks. Our baby was destroyed with "Baby Acne" which is a telltale of CMPI. This formula really helped with the dairy problem, did nothing for the reflux. That was another A&E trip and thankfully they prescribed Zantac which worked wonders for us!"

"We used Pepti 1 for a short while, but after an initial improvement he went downhill again. It was better when we added Colief, so that proved he was reacting to the small amount of lactose in it".

Aptamil, Pepti 2

This is nutritionally tailored to support a *cow's milk free* weaning diet. It contains a unique blend of GOS/FOS prebiotics and an extensively hydrolysed formula, which means that the cow's milk proteins have been extensively broken down. This makes Aptamil easier for babies to tolerate and consume whilst providing them with all the nutrition they need.

Parent's Review

"We use *Pepti 2 now with no problems. My fella stopped screaming the day I put him on it so it's been a lifesaver for us, it's the only thing that made any difference. A friend of mine whose baby had reflux gave me a tin of it. We had tried Nutramigen and C&G Anti-reflux before that to no avail".*

Aptamil, AR (Anti Reflux)

This is designed for the dietary management of frequent reflux and regurgitation. It is a nutritionally complete, thickened formula, which is

77

easy to digest. It contains LCPs (omega 3 & 6) and nucleotides suitable from birth.

Parent's Review

"I used Aptamil AR (anti-reflux/regurgitation) thicker feed, stays down. It definitely eased the reflux for two of my babies. Can't use Gaviscon with AR formula but I used to follow the directions for Gaviscon for a breastfed baby and syringe it in. You need to use largest teat size and watch for constipation with the AR formulas. Incidentally, I don't think you can get infant Gaviscon outside of Ireland and UK, could be wrong, but definitely not available here in UAE".

Cow & Gate, Pepti Junior

This formula, suitable from birth, is specially formulated with hydrolysed whey protein, and contains MCT **(medium chain triglycerides)** oil, which is easier to digest for babies with malabsorption or who need a milk-free diet.

Parent's Review

"Our baby was on Cow and Gate Anti-Reflux very thick, bottles completely stayed down, but once she started solids the regurgitation was back after food. It did make her quite constipated".

Nanny Care, Goat's Milk[17]

This is the highest quality milk from grass-fed New Zealand goats raised without stimulants and hormones. The milk is further fortified with vitamins, minerals and essential nutrients. Nutritionally, goat milk has certain physical properties in relation to its curd formation and fat characteristics which suggest that it can be more easily digested and is gentler on the digestive system. It contains different fat, protein & less lactose compared to cow's milk.

---

[17] Agency, F. S., Goats' milk formula, not a solution for cows' milk allergic infants. 2014. [Online]: Available at: http://www.food.gov.uk/news-updates/news/2014/6003/goats-milk#.U2DtuvldUko [Accessed 12 May 2014].

Parent's Review

"We used it for a while but after he had the antibiotics everything went pear-shaped and he started reacting to it. There was no actual evidence found to say that the use of the formula was any different to cow's milk formula. A baseline study [18] was carried out in 2012 where a number of babies were fed goat's milk infant formula and the other half breastfed but all tests showed that the babies fed goat's milk were no different development wise to those breastfed! I know there has been a change since as I spoke to the care line after Christmas and they said the European Food Safety Authority has now began to recognise Nanny Care infant formula as an alternative formula to cow's milk for use in infants. Nutritionally it contains everything the other formulas contain except DHA and ARA!"

See the References section for a link to the in-depth findings of the European Food Safety Authority in relation to goat's milk infant formula.

---

[18] European Food Safety Authority, Scientific Opinion on the suitability of goat milk protein as a source of protein in infant formulae and in follow-on formulae, EFSA Journal 2012;10(3):2603[18 pp.]. doi:10.2903/j.efsa.2012.2603.
Available at http://www.efsa.europa.eu/en/efsajournal/pub/2603.htm

It is important to note that the European Food Safety Authority (EFSA) has warned that goat's milk formula may not be suitable for infants with an allergy to cow's milk proteins. The proteins in cow's and goat's milk are so similar that a baby allergic to one would almost certainly be allergic to the other.

Enfamil, Ar. (Anti-Reflux)

Enfamil A.R. (Anti-Reflux) is a pre-thickened formula designed for infants with reflux. It is nutritionally complete and suitable for babies from birth onwards (term infants).

Parents' Reviews

"My little one is on the Enfamil Ar. formula with Colief (Anti colic) drops added. It is pre-thickened already and within a week on it she was keeping down the majority of her feeds. To help with the acid she was prescribed Zantac and once they got the dosage right between the formula and Zantac (ranitidine) she improved greatly. It does cause constipation though, so she needs Lactulose daily. She is 7 months now and will be on it for the foreseeable future".

81

"I used Enfamil Ar. for my baby and it worked wonders, it was the only formula that stayed down. It's thickened so with my Dr Brown bottles I had to use the Y flow teats so the formula flowed easily. I also found for my baby that using the standard bottle size lessened her gulping the formula which in turn reduced the reflux reactions i.e. hiccups, throwing up etc. On the Enfamil Ar. formula I found her poos were very stinky more so than usual poos, we thankfully had no constipation issues on this formula and my baby one was on it from 2 months to just over a year old and transitioned to cow's milk without much hassle".

SMA Staydown

This is a nutritionally complete formula for the dietary management of babies with significant reflux (regurgitation/spitting up) who are not being breastfed. It thickens in the tummy not in the bottle. It can be used as the sole source of nutrition from birth in place of your usual formula feed, and can be mixed with foods once weaning has begun.

Parents' Reviews

"We use SMA Staydown. It does just that, stays down. Regular milk was flowing up. Small amount still comes up but nothing like before. I gave up on Zantac. He hated it. Still a windy baby though. Water has to be fridge cold before you add formula".

"The Staydown and Anti-Reflux definitely causes constipation for us, our little man had severe reflux with aspiration and only Anti-Reflux with Losec helped control it".

Hypoallergenic Formula Non Prescription

Hypoallergenic formulas should never be used without a Doctors or Dieticians recommendation, and should only be used when there is a medical reason.

Nutramigen, Lipil 1 & 2

Nutramigen Formula – Proven to support visual development. Nutramigen LIPIL – over 68 years of managing infants with cow's milk allergy Nutramigen Lipil is a special, hypoallergenic formula for babies and children with cow's milk protein allergy or intolerance. Cow's milk allergy/intolerance may result in a variety of symptoms which may include eczema, colic, diarrhoea or constipation.

Nutramigen Lipil 1 is indicated for milk protein sensitivity, lactose intolerance, and galactosaemia and galactokinase deficiency. The protein in Nutramigen Lipil has been extensively broken down (hydrolysed) into tiny pieces that are not recognised by the immune system and will not trigger an allergic reaction in most infants. Nutramigen Lipil is lactose-free and is available as Nutramigen Lipil 1, which is suitable for babies from birth and Nutramigen Lipil 2, which is suitable from 6 months onwards and contains more calcium for older babies.

LIPIL is a special blend of nutrients, DHA and ARA, also known as Omega 3 and Omega 6 fatty acids.

DHA and ARA are present in breast milk and are important building blocks for a baby's brain and eyes. If your baby has a cow's milk allergy and difficulty absorbing fat your healthcare professional may recommend Pregestimil Lipil.

Raven was put on this formula at the initial stages of her CMSPI [19] journey. We found the first few days on this formula fine, but she soon developed a severe case of what resembled baby acne that continued to get worse by the day. She also developed a red ring around the perianal area of her bum and her eyes became very swollen and puffy. Raven was then moved onto an amino-based formula.

We have since discovered that she was having a reaction to the synthetic form of DHA and ARA [20] that is present in almost all baby formulas. Single cell oil DHA and ARA are extracted from laboratory-grown fermented algae and fungus and processed utilising a petroleum-derived hexane solvent. These oils manufactured are known as DHASCO and ARASCO (microbial oils rich in the long-chain polyunsaturated fatty acids), which are docosahexaenoic acid single cell oil and arachidonic acid single cell oil.

---

[19] GIKids, Digestive Topics: Cow's Milk Protein Intolerance, [Online] Available at: http://www.gikids.org/content/103/en/ [Accessed Feb2015]

[20] Vallaeys, Charlotte, *DHA and ARA in Infant Formula Dangerous and Unnecessary—Synthetic Additives Have No Place in Infant Foods* May 2010—

It is our belief that Raven could not tolerate these traces of the chemical hexane and her health improved dramatically when such food was removed.

You can read a full report provided on adverse reactions to DHA and ARA following The Cornucopia Institute[21] reference below.

It should also be noted that millions of babies from around the world have no reaction to the synthetic oils and can tolerate formula with DHA and ARA without any issues. Nevertheless, it is important to note that I and others in my group have found that such formulas caused a lot of problems in our babies.

Parents' Reviews

"I'm using the Polish brand of Nutramigen with the Lipil, which my pharmacy had started to stock; this contains no DHA or ARA. She was initially on Nutramigen Lipil 1 which contains DHA & ARA. She was on 10mgs of Losec and Carobel, also Gaviscon during a flare up. Within a month of starting the Polish made Nutramigen she came off Losec, Carobel and Gaviscon and is flying, suffers the very odd flare but I can manage it with a single sachet of Gaviscon in

---

[21] Will Fantle, T. C. I., 2008. DHA/ARA docosahexaenoic acid and arachidonic acid, The Cornucopia Institute, P.O. Box 126, Cornucopia, WI 54827: Will Fantle, The Cornucopia Institute

her feed for a few days. I also found that she was very sensitive to new food on the Lipil one, whereas now she can eat everything except milk and beef".

"Screaming, heightened reflux, congestion, facial markings (were the results). Screaming was so bad especially on Nutramigen AA and on Neocate that he was aspirating".

"Extremely windy baby. The Reflux flares constantly. I could see a huge improvement when moved to non-DHA formula. Less wind and normal bowel movements and reflux medication could be reduced".

"We used Nutramigen; the dietician recommended it to us after numerous other formulas. I think it was nearly 8 months into our nightmare reflux journey and with Losec it was amazing. Almost overnight our baby stopped screaming out in pain and sleeping a bit better. We then gradually introduced dairy to the diet after a few months and never looked back. I waited until he was 1 and a half before taking him off the formula and used ordinary milk as I was too scared for things to go backwards but it was fine".

"We used Nutramigen on my little girl, She had SR and was allergic to dairy, we tried so many different types of food till a paed doctor recommended Nutramigen. I think she was about 5 months. By

God what a change it was, she was 2 before we took her off it as were told she needed it over the dairy, we took her off it in April this year and slowly weaned her onto dairy and she's after growing out the allergy to dairy. She's now eating cheese, chocolate and other dairy things, still on soya milk as full milk didn't agree with her, then when my little boy was 6 weeks he was on Aptamil and started to go down these roads as my little girl and we put him straight onto Nutramigen and he's perfect since".

Hypoallergenic Amino Acid-Based Formulas

Are made from 100% non-allergenic amino acids and are only available on prescription, from your hospital or GP.

Nutramigen, AA Formula

Nutramigen AA Formula (amino acid) is an amino acid-based formula for babies with a severe cow's milk protein allergy or with multiple food allergies, who may not tolerate an extensively hydrolysed formula.

Unlike the hydrolysed formulas where cow's milk proteins are broken down during the manufacturing process, Nutramigen AA is made with 100% non-allergenic free amino acids, the building blocks of protein, so there are no cow's milk proteins whatsoever in this formula, therefore eliminating any risk of allergy.

We tried this formula and found that Raven's symptoms worsened as Nutramigen AA has a much higher percentage of DHA and ARA. Although it was not suitable for our baby, many parents from the group found this to be very beneficial to the health of their babies.

Parents' Reviews

"My baby's so much happier and settled on Nutramigen AA. She was on the Lipil version but it didn't really work. It is so expensive, twice the price of the Lipil version".

"We tried Nutramigen AA - disaster altogether and probably the worst reaction to all formulas we've tried. It was instant and he screamed the house down. I had never heard him scream like he did with it. I've since found out it contains high levels of DHA. WySoy caused a reaction with hives and reflux flare up (it also contains DHA) then we tried Infasoy (doesn't contain any DHA) and

we are still on it!! It's been a lifesaver for us as all amino acid-based formulas and hydrolysed ones were a no no!!! "

Neocate LCP

The proteins in *Neocate LCP* have been replaced with amino acids with the addition of long chain polyunsaturated (hence the name LCP) fatty acids, which have been demonstrated to assist with healthy brain and eye development and which may not be available in a restricted diet. The levels of these important LCPs in Neocate LCP closely match those found in breast milk and meet international guidelines for LCPs in infant formula.

Parents' Reviews

"GP recommended Nutramigen after a succession of formulas (nanny care, Aptamil Comfort, Aptamil). We found it only improved the reflux for an initial period of a couple of days and only slightly. The paed consultant put him on Neocate and he has improved hugely and is far more settled since".

"When we moved to Neocate at 15 weeks I saw a huge difference from Nutramigen but then once we started solids at nearly 7 months that rocked the boat for a long time. When he turned one we changed to Neocate Active with no DHA & his wind certainly improved a lot. Once he settled on Neocate Active we were able to wean off the Losec which went well after a rocky start. Wish I knew about Neocate from day one!!"

Neocate Advance / Neocate Junior

Neocate Advance is a nutritionally complete, amino acid-based powdered formula, designed to provide complete nutritional support or dietary supplementation for children with cow's milk allergy and multiple food protein intolerance. Neocate Advance is designed for children aged 1-10 years.

Although this is a formula for babies who are 12 months and over, this was given safely under medical supervision to Raven at four months old as it was the only amino-based formula that did not contain DHA or ARA. The batch of feed was diluted and one scoop of paediatric seravit was added to compensate for missing vitamins lost from the dilution.

We found this formula fantastic and could see immediate results. We could wean her off the dose of 25mg Losec a day and she remained off all meds until she turned 12 months old. I have since tried unsuccessfully to wean her totally back on to dairy.

Chapter 6

Alternative Remedies and Therapy

Giving a baby medication seems to be the last thing any parent wants to do. I have found in my experience that parents will exhaust all areas and try alternative solutions.

On our quest to fix Raven we have tried and tested a few and have also spent a small fortune. I have also drawn from the experience of parents from SRI group.

Faith Healing [22]

Definition: *recourse to divine power to cure mental or physical disabilities, either in conjunction with orthodox medical care or in place*

---

[22]   Encyclopaedia Britannica, *Faith healing;* Definition [Online] Available at http://www.britannica.com/EBchecked/topic/200569/faith-healing [Accessed Feb 2015]

of it. Often an intermediary is involved, whose intercession may be all-important in effecting the desired cure. Sometimes the faith may reside in a particular place, which then becomes the focus of pilgrimages for the sufferers.

Parents' Experiences

I have tried this myself; we contacted a lovely man to receive the "cure" this however did not work for us, although I have heard it being successful for other ailments in children".

"We went to one who told me my little boy would be fine in a few days. Two months later it was still the same".

"We went to one and our wee one hasn't looked back since".

"We visited 3 times with Sam and mild improvements but not loads but some people swear by it".

"We went to see one. We had to go 3 days and literally within a week the silent reflux was gone, no grunting, no arching her back absolutely nothing and she started sleeping through the night from then as well. That was when she was 10 1/2 weeks old and she's now 22 1/2 weeks! I really do believe in them as my mam is a curer of the whooping cough but like he said you don't need to

believe because your baby doesn't know the difference so it will work for them".

I lately ascertained that more and more parents are being required by some faith healers to cease their baby's medication and special dairy free formula prior to receiving the cure. In my opinion, this is not a safe practice and could actually create more issues for your baby. I always advise parents to seek medical advice when faced with these requests.

Kinesiology[23]

Definition: *Kinesiology is a series of tests that locate weaknesses in specific muscles reflecting imbalances throughout the body. Then specific massages or acupressure techniques are used in an attempt to rebalance what has been revealed by the kinesiology tests. Thus, kinesiology is used as both an assessment tool and as a limited therapeutic modality[24].*

Kinesiology claims to be a healing system that detects and corrects imbalances in the body before they develop into a disease, and which

---

[23] Farlex Partner Medical Dictionary, *Applied Kinesiology,* © Farlex 2012 [Online] Available at: http://medicaldictionary.thefreedictionary.com/applied+kinesiology [Accessed 20 April 2014].

[24] Farlex Partner Medical Dictionary, *Therapeutic modality.* (n.d.) *Jonas: Mosby's Dictionary of Complementary and Alternative Medicine.* (2005). [Online] Available at http://medical-dictionary.thefreedictionary.com/therapeutic+modality [Accessed April 2014]

restores overall system balance and harmony. It is used to alleviate muscle, bone, and joint problems, treat all manner of aches and pains, and correct many areas of imbalance and discomfort.

Parents' Experiences

"We found it to be the answer to our son's reflux. She suggested cutting down/ giving up wheat and dairy. This worked for him by cutting out wheat completely and just cutting out cow's milk. It also involved eating different foods to heal the gut but he won't really eat all of these foods, for example, pineapple and beetroot. He does eat berries though! Add lemon juice to water. Eat more plants. Drink stock/ soup from boiling bones. Eat only good quality meat".

"Went to a kinesiologist and were told to take him off dairy, wheat, sugar and cauliflower (something we would have eaten at least twice a week). Definitely a turning point for us."

NAET Therapy[25]

NAET (Nambudripad's Allergy Elimination Techniques)

By definition: Allergy Elimination is a gentle & non-invasive therapy for treating the body for food and environmental allergies. NAET has been available in the United States for over 30 years and is a well-known treatment; it has only become available in Ireland recently.

[26]*"Your NAET practitioner will take a case history of any previous illnesses, medical conditions and/or symptoms. Then, using kinesiology, chiropractic and acupressure techniques, your practitioner will balance the energy of your body to the allergies and intolerances that have been causing discomfort and interfering with your wellbeing. NAET is not a 'quick fix'. It is performed at weekly or monthly intervals, depending on the client's needs. NAET will help with bloating, headaches, hay fever, gluten and dairy intolerance, skin conditions and other general pains and body aches. Most unexplained symptoms of pain or discomfort can be*

---

[25] Nambudripad, Devi S. (2003). NAET: Say Goodbye to Asthma: A Revolutionary Treatment for Allergy-Based Asthma and Other Respiratory Disorders. Say Good-Bye To... Series. Delta Publishing Company. p.37Wikipedia 2014 Nambudripad's Allergy Elimination Techniques (NAET), http://en.wikipedia.org/wiki/Nambudripad's_Allergy_Elimination_Techniques

[26] Bowman, H Naet-Europe [Online] Available at http://www.naet-_europe.com/en [Accessed May 17th 2014]

traced back to the body having an intolerant reaction to a substance, whether in contact, injected, ingested, or inhaled.

Once the body has been treated with NAET, clients find that they can then eat foods that previously caused them problems and remain symptom free. NAET is suitable for all ages, from new-borns with reflux problems due to cow's milk allergy, to children with asthma and people of all ages with unexplained health problems. It has also been used very successfully on children with autism and ADHD. NAET can help everyone. It truly is a wonderful system".

NAET is still under review in terms of independent substantiated evidence and there is continuing debate throughout the literature on its potential effectiveness[28]. Despite the lack of hard evidence on NAET, a lot of parents find it very helpful.

Acupuncture[27]

Definition: The practice of inserting needles into the body to reduce pain or induce anaesthesia. Acupuncture is a form of treatment for children and it has a long and respected history in China.

---

[27] MedicineNet, Inc. , 1996-2014. Definition of Acupuncture . [Online] Available at: http://www.medicinenet.com/script/main/art.asp?articlekey=2132 [Accessed Feb 2015]

"In Ireland, acupuncture is used in the treatment of babies and young kids but parents are often reluctant to bring their children for Traditional Chinese Medicine[28] (TCM) treatments even though the parents themselves have tried it before. They think that maybe the child is too young to benefit from it and also because kids tend to be afraid of needles.

In China, it is very common to use acupuncture to treat children as a preventive medicine as well as for childhood problems".

Parents' Experiences:

"We brought our baby to see one of these specialists, the specialist tapped areas on him related to his digestive system with what resembled a tiny hammer. Then put a plaster on his tummy to wear for a few days on a pressure point. To be honest this has really worked as he is completely off all meds now. I would have been very sceptical as I haven't brought him to any other treatments other than medical as I thought that was the best thing to do. But in hindsight I wished I had brought him here 1st as it would have saved 3 years of sleepless nights and tears

---

[28] MedicineNet, Inc. , 1996-2014. Definition of Acupuncture. [Online] Available at: http://www.medicinenet.com/script/main/art.asp?articlekey=2132 [Accessed Feb 2015]

both ours and his. On saying that, I am still keeping his appointments with the hospital and the dietician. Using a bit of both worlds".

Osteopathy[29]

Definition: *Osteopathy is a way of detecting, treating and preventing health problems by moving, stretching and massaging a person's muscles and joints.*

Osteopathy is based on the principle that the wellbeing of an individual depends on their bones, muscles, ligaments and connective tissue functioning smoothly together. Osteopaths believe their treatments allow the body to heal itself. They use a range of techniques but do not use drugs or surgery.

---

29 Murray, Rhona, MPSI, BSc. Pharm Hons Biochemistry M.An.Sc., Health A-Z , Homepharm. [Online] Available at http://www.homepharm.ie/index.php?route=information/nhs/nhs2&id=Osteopathy [Accessed Feb 2015]

Parents' Experiences

"I brought my little one to the osteopath when she was 6 weeks old. He cured her hiccupping as he said her diaphragm was distorted from having them but told me that he wouldn't be much use to her for reflux. We brought her to a chiropractor at 4.5 months. Didn't see any change in her after 3 visits so stopped going".

"I went to an osteopath and after two sessions he honestly found a switch in her that stopped the crying. It was seriously life changing in our house. I would have tried anything but another mother swore by this guy to me and it made a huge difference".

"We did 7 sessions with an osteopath and no improvement, only turning point was going on Neocate; don't think anything works unless food and medication are right. After taking him to faith healer at 8 months we were able to take him off meds! Due again in June and if this baby is the same we'll definitely go to him if he's still there! I'd be willing to try anything not to go through the same again!!"

Cranio-Sacral Therapy[30]

Definition: *"Cranio-sacral Therapy (CST) is a light-touch hands-on therapy that enhances the body's natural capacity for healing. It is a gentle form of manipulation, Cranio-sacral therapy (CST) is a hands-on healing technique typically practiced by physical therapists, massage therapists, and chiropractors. Cranio-sacral therapists manipulate the Cranio-sacral system, which includes the soft tissue and bones of the head (cranium), the spine down to its tail end (the sacral area), and the pelvis. They also work with the membranes that surround these bones and the cerebro-spinal fluid that bathes the brain and spinal cord. Although the therapist uses a touch so light that many patients don't even notice it, most people report feeling profoundly relaxed after a treatment."*

Parents' Experiences

"I did Cranio-sacral therapy and baby massage and I found that both helped a bit - def some of the massage technique helps when it is bad at night".

---

[30]. Irish Association of Craniosacral Therapists, *What is Craniosacral Therapy*, [online] Available at http://iacst.ie/craniosacral-therapy. [Accessed Feb 2015]

"Found cranial osteopathy great for constipation. Really works for a few days after but not for reflux".

"Cranio-sacral worked re hiccups, constipation etc. but not much for reflux".

"We did craniosacral therapy and I did find it good. It didn't stop his reflux but she worked on me, the hubby and the baby and honestly - something changed. We had three sessions and what I found was that because of everything that was happening with the baby, trying and fighting for answers, the exhaustion, bickering, worry, stress etc. it helped 'ground' us all again. It definitely helped settle him a bit and it did me the world of good too".

Chiropractic Adjustment

Definition: *"Chiropractic adjustment[31] is a procedure in which trained specialists (chiropractors) use their hands or a small instrument to apply a controlled, sudden force to a spinal joint. The goal of chiropractic*

---

[31] Chiropractic First Dublin, Jan 2015, *Chiropractic Adjustment.* [Online] Available at:
     http://www.chiropracticfirstdublin.ie/index.php/chiropractic/ [Accessed Feb 2015]

adjustment, also known as spinal manipulation, is to correct structural alignment and improve your body's physical function."

We used one of these ourselves for Raven in the early days. The practitioner said her alignment was off because my labour went fast towards the end of an 18 hour delivery. He made a few adjustments and we attended his practice three times, but it made no difference to her health at all.

Parents' Experiences

"We went to a chiropractor and it helped get rid of the hiccups she was getting all the time but that's it".

"We found our chiropractor great for colic but it did not seem to ease the reflux at all, there was an improvement in bowel movements for some time. Sessions are quite expensive but as you know a worried parent will try everything to help their child".

Chapter 7

Herbal & Non-Prescription Products

Colic Calm

"Homeopathic remedies can be an excellent choice for treating infant colic symptoms. Homeopathy is safe and completely allergen-free and side-effect-free. There is only one such liquid formula on the market.

Colic Calm Gripe Water is available at leading pharmacies, online and in selected health food stores and health practitioners' offices. Colic Calm has a success rate of over 90% in treating baby colic. Many parents and caretakers have been relieved to find an all-natural remedy. The unique homeopathic formula works within minutes, so it is only given on an "as needed" basis. Thousands of satisfied customers have also reported that it works wonders for bloating, pressure, stomach cramps, hiccups, teething and even acid reflux. It is also extremely effective on gas created during introduction of new foods into babies' delicate digestive tracts.

A combination of homeopathic ingredients is used to treat the multiple symptoms of colic"[32].

We loved Colic Calm. While it did not do much for Raven's reflux, as hers was very severe, it did help with the colic she developed at six weeks. It also helped her to sleep. I still give it now and it helps with her hiccups. I liked the fact that it was natural. She also seemed to like the taste too. Only problem is, it is black and can stain the clothes, so be careful giving it.

Herbal Remedies

"The pharmaceutical drugs used by doctors today are derived from the plants traditionally used by herbalists. Using these plants in the traditional way is gentler on the body as they work in harmony with the body's natural ability to heal itself.

Unfortunately, not all ailments can be fully cured, but where we cannot cure the ailment, we strive to make life more comfortable by reducing the pain or other symptoms of the underlying condition.

---

[32] Ketomi Distribution, Colic Calm @2013-2014. *Colic Calm*. [Online] Available at: http://www.coliccalm.com.au/blog/cat/baby-colic-gas-reflux [Accessed 12 April 2014].

Dunboyne Herbs is located on the outskirts of Dublin, just off the M50 on an organic farm in the countryside of County Meath. Our team of growers and herbalists produce a wide range of natural herbal products on site. Dunboyne Herbs have skilled, expert herbalists from around the country. The knowledge, empathy and professionalism of these experts have contributed to the Dunboyne Herbs' reputation as one of the leading herbal clinics in the country.

In addition to its herbal therapists, Dunboyne Herbs have a variety of other professionals working as part of a multidisciplinary team. This team is skilled in Sports rehabilitation, Sports massage therapy, Yoga, Amatsu and Reiki. At Dunboyne Herbs we provide a wide range of treatments that allow us to provide a holistic approach to health and well-being" [33]

When we weaned Raven off Losec (Omeprazole; see Chapter 8) at four months we used herbs which consisted of *Chrysanthemum leucanthemum* and *Equisetum arvense*. We found them fantastic. I would highly recommend this practice, especially for parents with babies who have GOR or colic.

---

[33] Mc Goldrick, Dorothy, Commonly Treated conditions, Colic in Babies, Dunboyne Herbs. Information available at http://www.dunboyneherbs.ie

Parent View: Mother of Twins with Reflux

"All in all they are both doing really well and benefiting from the herbs. And given I have two with reflux, one particularly bad, and see improvements says a lot. Definitely this is worth a try for some of you".

Cow and Gate Instant Carobel

Carobel and Xanthan gum (for readers from outside Ireland) are specially designed for medical purposes and can be spoon-fed as a paste or directly added to liquids. Instant Carobel is for use in the dietary management of habitual and recurrent vomiting, dysphagia and rumination. Cow and Gate Instant Carobel is suitable for full-term infants, children and adults. Carobel (135 g) may be added to an infant's milk or drink (water/juice), or given by spoon as a thick gel just prior to drinking, or eating a very wet meal.

Used as a spoon-feed or paste:

This method is appropriate for breastfed infants and may be the preferred method for bottle-fed infants. It is also suitable for first weaning foods that have too liquid a consistency and for older children and adults.

We found this great for thickening Raven's feeds as, the formula we used had a thin consistency. It is tricky to master at the start and it takes trial and error to get the consistency right. The longer the feed is left the thicker it gets. I lost count of the amount of teats we had to throw out as we tried to make the holes bigger ourselves. We also found this made Raven very constipated.

Gaviscon, Baby Gaviscon

"Gaviscon Infant helps to prevent gastric regurgitation in infants where competence of the cardiac sphincter (the valve between the distal end of the oesophagus and the stomach) has not been fully established.

The indications for use are gastric regurgitation, gastro-oesophageal reflux and reflux associated with hiatus hernia in infants and young children.

It should not to be used in premature infants or infants under one year except under medical supervision. It is for oral use after mixing with water or milk feeds.

Gaviscon Infant contains two active ingredients, sodium alginate and magnesium alginate. These are naturally occurring substances that are found in a particular type of seaweed. Alginates[34] act locally in the stomach to physically prevent the contents of the stomach from flowing back into the food pipe (reflux) and being regurgitated."

Unfortunately Gaviscon Infant did nothing for Raven and made her very constipated; it seems to work well for babies with a milder form of reflux or GOR. It also seems to be used as a first port of call by doctors and can be successful.

Probiotics

Dr Martha Koehn[35] has kindly allowed me to use this adaptation from her online blog:

"Some babies, who are born by C-section, are on antibiotics, get no colostrum, or all of the above, and are not necessarily doomed

---

[34] The National Magazine Company Ltd, 2014. NetDoctor.co.uk - The UK's leading independent health website. [Online] Available at: http://www.netdoctor.co.uk/ [Accessed 04 May 2014]

[35] Koehn, M., 2011. Help for Acid Reflux, Heartburn, GERD, Indigestion, IBS, Gastro paresis, and Many Other Digestive Issues. [Online] Available at: http://help4acidreflux.wordpress.com/ [Accessed 28 June 2014]

for digestive problems. Some babies are really strong and healthy and their body has no problems making and building up its own probiotics. But for some, this can be the start of the digestive system not working well.

Most babies will greatly benefit from a probiotic supplement. When someone is low on probiotics, they are low on many, so the best supplement would be one that has at least 10 different strains in it. But the bottom line is that your child gets relief.

Many children with digestive problems can have a lack of sufficient digestive enzymes. Digestive enzymes are what are in all foods (before they are cooked or processed) to aid in breaking them down. They are especially needed for breaking down proteins. If a nursing mom eats a diet of mostly raw foods this can help some but unless the foods are organically grown, they are not very enzyme rich. The pancreas is what makes digestive enzymes and it will try to compensate for the lack of them in foods, but for some babies it can be difficult for their pancreas to keep up making enough to break down the food (proteins in particular) that they take in whether it be through breast milk, formula, or solids as they get older.

It is possible for a baby to inherit the problem of the pancreas not being capable of producing enough digestive enzymes, and for these children, they may carry this problem all of their life. Very similar to the diabetic, who cannot make enough insulin.

When "food" is placed in the stomach, the stomach will excrete a small amount of acid to activate the enzymes so they will start breaking down the food. If there are no or little enzymes, then the stomach will excrete a little more acid. Eventually the food is forced into the intestines even if it isn't fully properly broken down. If the food isn't broken down then it will be very difficult for the body to be able to absorb and use it. For some children, this undigested food will sit in the intestines too long and the longer "food" stays in the intestines, the more moisture that is drawn out of it, and it can cause constipation.

This excess acid that the stomach makes can play a major part in some babies' digestive problems. Too much acid will kill probiotics. And as probiotics are the protective coating for the entire digestive tract, then without it, the food, reflux, or stool will rub right up next to the oesophagus and intestines and can cause them to become raw, inflamed, and even bleed sometimes.

So, how have digestive enzymes and probiotics affected my children? Well, they have made a HUGE difference. Cure? No. They have been taking a supplement of them for 2 years and today they are able to eat any and all foods. But they have to take a pill with every meal and any snack that does not have enzymes in it. I still try not to let my boys have a lot of dairy though. But if they ask for a glass of milk I normally let them. They were not used to drinking milk when they were younger so it is not something they like terribly well. One evening a while ago, when I let them have a glass of milk, I reminded them to take a pill with it. I put them to bed, read those stories, and then sat in there for a few minutes with them. After Quinton fell asleep, I noticed how restless he was. Soon he sat fully up he was so uncomfortable but he didn't wake up. This reminded me so much of how he used to be and I got to thinking that he had probably not taken a pill. So I went and got 2 of them with a glass of water and woke him up and made him take them. I was impressed how in about a minute he completely settled down and peacefully slept the rest of the night.

After seeing how the probiotics and enzymes helped my children so much, some of my fear started to leave of having another baby with digestive problems. I started taking probiotics and enzymes as part of my prenatal vitamins. (You can read more about my baby that is acid reflux free our healthy 3rd child).

And how have probiotics and digestive enzymes helped me? Well, a little TMI but I used to be constipated and suffer from haemorrhoids pretty much all the time. After about 3 months of taking the supplement I realized that I was "going" every day and also my haemorrhoids were much better! Eventually they disappeared and have only returned once for a short while after I had my baby. As for constipation it pretty much stays at bay unless I get careless in taking the pills. I have also been very pleased at how seldom I get bloated and rarely have stomach aches like I used to so often. A cure-all? Again, no but VERY beneficial!!

There are many different brands and companies out there that sell probiotic and enzyme supplements. We use a product called "Digestive Health" sold by core health products. It contains 13 different strains of pH stabilized probiotics, prebiotics (which are food for the probiotics); over 20 types of broad spectrum plant based digestive enzymes, and several different types of soothing herbs. I personally recommend using Digestive Health because I know that is what has worked for me and many others, but if you wish to look for a different brand then go to how to choose the right probiotic/enzyme supplements.

If you decide to try probiotics and/or enzymes, be aware that it can possibly make symptoms worsen for a day or two. This is called Herxheimer Reaction[36]

---

[36] Chronic Illness Recovery Counsel Liaison Education, Herxheimer Reaction, [Online] Available at: https://chronicillnessrecovery.org/index.php?option=com_content&view=article&id=161 [Accessed Feb 2015]

Chapter 8

Prescription Medications

Drug Classes and Mechanisms

Ranitidine[37] (Zantac)

"Ranitidine is an oral drug that blocks the production of acid by acid-producing cells in the stomach. It belongs to a class of drugs called H2 (histamine-2) blockers, that also includes cimetidine (Tagamet), nizatidine (Axid) and famotidine (Pepcid).

Histamine is a naturally-occurring chemical that stimulates cells in the stomach (parietal cells) to produce acid. H2-blockers inhibit the action of histamine on the cells, thus reducing the production of acid by the stomach. Since excessive stomach acid can damage the oesophagus,

---

[37] MedicineNet, Inc., 1996-2014. Ranitidine, Zantac: Drug Facts, Side Effects and Dosing. [Online] Available at: http://www.medicinenet.com/ranitidine/article.htm [Accessed 17 March 2014].

stomach, and duodenum and lead to inflammation and ulceration, reducing stomach acid prevents and heals acid-induced inflammation and ulcers. The FDA approved Ranitidine in October 1984[38]".

The brand name Zantac comes in a liquid form for babies. Zantac has been known to give brilliant results for many babies with reflux. Zantac is dosed according to babies' weight, and it is therefore advised by doctors that the dose is increased as the baby gains weight. It should be stored in a cool dry place away from heat and moisture and discarded after four weeks as it loses its potency.

Many parents claim it is hard to get their babies to take Zantac as the taste is very sour; giving it with gripe water seems to help. If you are still finding it hard to give via syringe, try to put the dose in the teat of your baby's bottle and give it that way. Zantac can be given before or after food.

Raven was prescribed Zantac after her first stay in hospital. She has silent reflux but this seemed to make her vomit, she actually threw up for a whole week. It was then decided she could not tolerate it and we moved to Losec (Omeprazole, see below).

---

[38] Heal Pharmacy, *Zantac (Ranitidine) generic* [Online] Available at http://www.healpharmacy.com/zantac-ranitidine-150-032-180-pills-p-5472.html. [Accessed Feb 2015]

Proton-Pump Inhibitors (PPIs)

Proton-Pump Inhibitors (PPIs) reduce the production of acid by blocking the enzyme in the wall of the stomach that produces acid. The reduction of acid prevents ulcers and allows any ulcers that exist in the oesophagus, stomach, and duodenum to heal.

Are There Differences among Proton Pump Inhibitors (PPIs)?

PPIs are very similar in action although there are some reports in scientific literature that suggests that esomeprazole (Nexium) is more potent that omeprazole. Although all PPIs have similar mechanisms they are different chemically so they may differ in potency. What might be lacking in this area are well designed comparative studies to get a clear picture on how these PPIs measure up against each other.

Many parents will say their baby did better when a specific PPI was changed. Raven did not do too good on Losec and could tolerate Zoton better. They differ in how they are broken down by the liver and their drug interactions. The effects of some PPIs may last longer and therefore, may be taken less frequently.

There are many brands of PPI on the market used worldwide under different names:

1. Lansoprazole, (Solu tab, Zoton, Prevacid),
2. Omeprazole, (Losec, Mups, Prilosec, Zegerid contains omerprazole and sodium bicarbonate),
3. Rabeprazole (Aciphex)
4. Pantoprazole (Protonix)
5. Esomeprazole (Nexium)

The dosage for a PPI is often calculated based on the weight of the baby, although many doctors will prescribe a standard dose. When PPIs are dosed according to weight, the dosage may need be altered over time to reflect growth of the baby. Never increase the dose of your baby's medication without the consent of a doctor or paediatrician.

As I am from Ireland, I can only make reference to the two main brands that are used here to treat children, which are *Losec Mups* (AstraZeneca UK Limited, active ingredient Omeprazole) *and Zoton* (Pfizer, active ingredient Lansoprazole).

Our experience with administering adult medication to a tiny baby was a minefield of trial and error. There is also a liquid Losec formulation available, but it is very expensive and is known to lose its potency after two weeks.

We received a lot of conflicting advice for administering *Losec* from pharmacists and doctors. I performed a great deal of research on the best ways to give it and how.

I found our friends across in the United Sates were so ahead in terms of reflux awareness and the associated medications.

Anyone who has a baby with reflux disease will go to the ends of the earth to try help their baby. I remember countless nights trawling through websites looking for answers. I established that the medical field do not see or grasp the devastation this can cause a family. I learned a good saying that a mother with a reflux child will do more investigation than the FBI!

One of the websites I found absolutely amazing was a site called *MARCI-Kids*, which is sadly no longer usable.

MARCI-Kids were owned by the University of Missouri. It was inspired by the research of Dr Jeffrey Phillips and Dr Marcella Bothwell, San Diego Children's Hospital (MARCI).

The *MARCI-Kids* site was dedicated to providing information to the caregivers of infants suffering from acid reflux, or suspected of having acid-related disorders. It provided valid information on treatment to assist the caregivers of infants who have acid reflux.

Dr Jeffrey Phillips is Director of research, and also the inventor of *Zegrid* (the adult PPI medication). Dr Phillips, referred to as Doctor P throughout, is board-certified as a Pharmacotherapy Specialist. His research concentrates on the development of drugs for treating gastric-acid related disorders such as stress ulcers in critically ill patients and gastro-esophageal and extra-esophageal reflux disease in paediatric patients. Dr. Phillips holds three patents, the most recent being for *Zegerid*, an immediate release, oral proton pump inhibitor formulation that is licensed to and marketed by *Santarus*, a San Diego-based specialty pharmaceutical company.

There would seem to be two different modes of action for different types of PPI. Delayed release PPIs and Immediate release PPIs. The practical differences, in terms of use for effective treatment, are explained below.

What I learned From Dr P – in Simple Terms

The acid pumps (called proton pumps), in acid making cells (called parietal cells) in the stomach, make acid when signalled to do so. They are signalled to make acid when you begin eating (mainly by food or milk). This lowers the pH in the stomach. After an evening meal the pumps go dormant till approx. 2am, when they become active and generate a large amount of acid. This pumping continues until approximately 7am.

The explanation for this is simple and genetic. In prehistoric times there was little in terms of cleanliness in preparing food and we humans did not cook well. There were no stoves, often not even fire, and food was often eaten raw. The largest meal of the day was eaten in the early evening (before 7pm) and after eating humans went to sleep. During the night acid pumps in the systems of these early humans became very active and made a lot of acid. This gave them the advantage of the acid killing any bacteria which may have been ingested during the meal. Successfully surviving the night and digesting the meal meant that the species thrived. This remnant genetic predisposition is still with us and we modern humans still have that 2am to 7am acid activity or *acid dump*.

This helps explain why Doctor Jeffrey Phillips[39] recommended giving Losec on an empty stomach 30mins before feeds, or 90mins after. He also suggested giving the last dose at 5.30pm as the acid pumps switch off at 7pm. Doctor P explains how and why it is important to give a PPI before 5.30 p.m.

---

[39] Zoom Info, *Dr. Jeffrey Phillips, Research Associate professor, University of Missouri-Columbia*, [Online] Available at http://www.zoominfo.com/p/Jeffrey-Phillips/81631039. [Accessed Feb 2015]

The Following Information is From Literature That Doctor P has Provided:

*"SoluTab, (zoton for my European readers) and any of the **Delayed release PPIs** do not work at night-time very well. Let me clarify.*

What does PPIs require to work? - Acid pumps in the stomach to be actively secreting acid.

How long is the PPI in your baby's system? - Approximately 120 minutes (2hrs) after you give it

From 9pm until about 2am there is very little acid production (this is ancient genetic encoding in humans). If acid pumps (proton pumps) are not active during the time period (0-2hrs) after drug treatment, then acid will not be blocked by the drug.

*If you give the **Delayed release PPI,** Prevacid, it will be in the baby's body for only 3.5/4 hrs after administration, and then it will dissipate and be unavailable.*

Therefore Prevacid PPI given after 5.30pm will have no effect because no active acid secreting cells will be pumping during the time the drug is in the bloodstream (0-2hrs after a 5.30pm treatment would be ineffective after 7pm).

- **_Immediate release PPIs_** such as Zegerid, or PPI mixed with Caracare (not available in Ireland) can be given without regard to meals (or even in the bottle) and can be given at any time day or night.

Immediate-release PPIs have a buffer that stimulates those pumps to come on (naturally active from 2 am till 7am) and then blocks them while they are on" (the buffer is also protecting the PPI from acid degradation). Remember the body shuts down its pumps after 7pm and stays shut down until approx 2am.

When you use a buffer and **_Immediate-Release_** PPI - the buffer hits the stomach and raises the pH. This makes the stomach lining send a signal to the acid secreting cells (parietal cells) to wake the pumps and get some of them making acid just as the PPI hit the pumps and shuts them down. When you use a buffer, a lot of these pumps get used up. Therefore, by giving a dose around 8 or 9pm, or thereabouts, the pumps are exhausted and there aren't any to come on in the 2am period - so then there is no acid dump.

PPI drugs (such as SoluTab) can only block pumps that are in place and ready to make acid. The acid pumps are finite (meaning there are only so many available in a 24 hour. Period).

Night-time Acid Issues: Acid Dump

We have a period of acid dump from 2am till about 7am. This is the period of maximal acid dump at night.

*Let's say you time it perfectly and give the dose (**Delayed release PPI**) 30mins after midnight (00.30am). The drug would be in absorption for a further 1.5hrs. At 2.00am (00.5hrs + 1.5 hrs absorption) the treatment begins to be effective and will continue for a further 2hrs until 4.00am. After 4.00am the drug has been lost from the system, but your body is still making loads of acid (nocturnal acid) until approximately 7.00am.*

This means that from 4.00am there is no protection from acid.

The other thing you should know is a Little PPI Pharmacology

"PPIs can only turn off <u>active</u> acid pumps. Therefore if the pumps are not on/active (in the resting phase) and you take a PPI (that does not have a buffer) then the PPI will simply get absorbed. This is because when PPI gets to the parietal cell, it finds no <u>active</u> acid pumps, and therefore cannot shut off any (<u>active</u>) pumps. In this case the now useless PPI will be removed through

normal metabolism and elimination (just as all drugs are removed from the body).

The studies were performed (not by me) to monitor the baseline pH (before treatment) and then after treatment. This baseline data proved the night-time (2-7am) acid dump"

I found this Information extremely helpful and it made total sense to give the PPI before 5:30 p.m.

Doctor P also states that the *PPI* must not be crushed and given with food, if a baby will not take it with water, use baby food puree or an acid-based substance, to dissolve the tablet.

I found useful information from a company called *Infant Acid Reflux Solutions* [40] they provide a solution called *BellyBuffers* and *TummyCare Max*. These products make a PPI **immediate release**, so there is no timing around feeding.

At the beginning of our reflux journey and during our initial experience with *Losec*, we learned the hard way. It is not the liquid from dissolving the tablet that is the important part of the medication; it is the beads that are left behind. I call them the magic beads!

---

[40] Infant Acid Reflux Solutions, *TummyCare Max* and *BellyBuffers* [Online] Available at: http://www.infant-acid-reflux-solutions.com [Accessed Feb 2015]

We eventually found ways of giving Raven her medication. We also split the overall dose and administered it twice a day, as a baby's metabolism works way faster than an adult's.

At first we tried using a large syringe. We popped the tablet inside and then drew up five millilitres of liquid and let the tablet dissolve. I then squirted it towards the back of the throat while blowing on her face (as this causes a swallowing response in babies). I found we never got all the beads when using the syringe. So we resorted to dissolving the tablet in a small med cup and pouring it onto a small medicine spoon. I would keep mixing this until I got all the beads and I would rub the remaining beads on the inside of her cheeks. I would then give her some water to wash it down.

A video of this can be found in my app Infant Acid Reflux available on iTunes and Google play to download to your device.

The "Acid Battle"

An important fact that doctors did not tell us about was the "acid battle" that follows giving a PPI for the first time. Parents can actually think that the PPI is making things worse.

Acid battle is when the PPI gets into the system and starts to shut off stomach pumps in the stomach to help reduce acid. The body responds by turning different pumps on whilst this is happening to counteract pumps being switched off. Basically the PPI is trying to turn off all the pumps, but not all pumps are on all the time, they come on in shifts. This results in a battle of the two. The body tries to fight the PPI by producing more acid to compensate, as it is not a natural thing to have reduced acid in the stomach.

The "battle" can continue for roughly ten days, and then it calms down.

Your Doctor may advise giving *Zantac* at this time and many parents have found this helpful, until the body adjusts to the new medication. Don't give up.

Acid Rebound Weaning off a PPI

PPIs are fantastic and can help so much, but it is important to note that long-term use of a PPI can have its problems. Suppressing the natural acid levels in the stomach can cause issues along the way.

When Raven was four months old, she contracted *Clostridium difficile* (C. Diff) which is a bacterium infection that can affect the digestive system. Symptoms can range from diarrhea to serious and potentially fatal inflammation of the colon.

There have been a many research studies which suggest that this can be one of the side effects of long-term use of a PPI[41]. The reduction of acid within the stomach can make it easier for bacteria to flourish and cause infection. Doctors will regularly ask parents to try to wean their babies off a PPI to see if the reflux symptoms have subsided. If at any stage it is recommended that you wean your baby off any PPI it is important to know about the process and what to expect.

Acid rebound can occur when the proton pump inhibitor (PPI) is stopped or weaned. Rebound symptoms are caused by the stomach adjusting to ceasing medication. The body is adding acid producing pumps regularly in response to receiving acid blocking medications.

When the medication ceases these pumps are still being turned on. This results in an overproduction of acid and Rebound symptoms. Many babies will experience this surge of acid when the PPI is stopped or weaned. Naturally many parents mistake this as a fail and put their

---

[41] Smith A. MD, Proton Pump Inhibitors and Clostridium Difficile Infection, March 20, 2014. [Online] Available at: http://www.clinicalcorrelations.org/?p=7409. [Accessed Feb 2015]

babies back on the medication at this point. However, these symptoms do pass if you allow the stomach time to adjust. When weaning, try to hang on in there and don't give up. Acid rebound can take up to 7 days for the effects of the PPI to leave the body.

If after Day 10 there are still symptoms of reflux, it is considered a fail and a PPI may be re-started. Pain relief for the baby is advised during the weaning process.

I remember the first time we weaned Raven down from 25mg of *Losec* when she was 4 months old. It was an absolute nightmare as she was in so much pain I had to use infant pain relief. If I had not been aware that this could happen and we could experience the rebound effect, I would most definitely have put her back on the medication. Nevertheless, on day 8 of the medication being stopped Raven stopped screaming and was fine for many months afterwards.

Ketotifen: Generic Name: Liquid Oral (Key-Toe-TIFF-En)

Ketotifen is an antihistamine used, usually in children, to help prevent or reduce the symptoms of asthma (e.g. Shortness of breath). Taken every day, it may also help reduce the severity and length of these symptoms.

It works by blocking a chemical (histamine) that may lead to swelling (inflammation) of the airways in the lungs.

Although *Ketotifen*'s primary use is to treat asthma in children it also is known to heal the gut. Babies who have had intolerance to dairy and soy in the past will almost always will have issues due to inflammation when it is time to wean onto solids.

On ingestion of the food, the child usually has many non-Immunoglobulin (IgE) mediated delayed symptoms such as congestion, sneezing, heightened reflux, facial marking and/or swelling, diarrhoea/constipation. These non-IgE reactions are caused when the mast cells in the body produce too much histamine.

Ketotifen blocks the cells from producing the histamine and in turn, heals and calms the gut. It will also help with appetite and aid sleep in children with severe Intolerance to foods.

Ketotifen & Intestinal Permeability

"I have been using the medication Ketotifen (oral suspension) with good results. Children's parents and some adults taking it as well report more normal bowel movements, less gas and bloating and decreased food reactions. Most of the time it seems to take

at least two to three weeks to notice these differences, but you should expect long-term use and immediate results may not be seen. A trial period of 60 days is recommended. Be patient and give it time to do its thing, which is to reduce intestinal inflammation and promote healing of a leaky gut" [42].

Raven is now on Ketotifen, the initial results were amazing and she ate and slept really well, this seemed to taper off and her appetite became sporadic. However over time her sleeping totally adjusted and she slept the night right through.

Recently Under our Doctor's supervision, we attempted to wean Raven off Ketotifen, the results were immediate, her food intake dropped dramatically and she lost weight in the weeks to follow, her behaviour became extremely erratic and her sleep pattern became totally out of sync again.

She is currently back to her usual dose and sleeping well; she has good and bad days where eating is concerned, personally I would totally

---

[42] Woelle, D. K., 2011, the official website of Doctor Kurt Woelle. [Online] Available at: http://drwoeller.com/ [Accessed 20 May 2014].

recommend Ketotifen for babies and children with intolerance and allergy to food.

I found with most medications that in the initial period of treatment, the improvements were great. Then for some unknown reason the baby may regress. I don't know why this happens, but this occurrence has been noted by a lot of parents.

You think you have cracked the disease and are coming down the home stretch; you give a sigh of relief and start to relax and enjoy your baby. Then suddenly you find yourself back to square one within days or weeks. I think this is one of the cruellest parts of the disease and it is very hard to deal with.

Chapter 9

Prokinetics/ Motility Drugs

Motility Drugs for Delayed Gastric Emptying

Prokinetics [43]

"Prokinetic agents, or prokinetics, are medications that help control acid reflux. Prokinetics help strengthen the lower oesophageal sphincter (LES) and cause the contents of the stomach to empty faster. This allows less time for acid reflux to occur.

Today, prokinetics are typically used with other gastro-oesophageal reflux disease (GORD) or heartburn medications, such as proton pump inhibitors (PPIs) or H2 receptor blockers. Unlike these other acid reflux medications, which all generally are safe, prokinetics may have serious or

---

[43] Healthline Networks, Inc., 2005-2014. *Pro-kinetic Agents: Bethanechol, Cisapride, Domperidone, and Metoclopramide.* [Online] Available at:
http://www.healthline.com/health/gerd/prokinetics#2 [Accessed 21 June 2014].

even dangerous side effects. They are often only used in the most serious cases of GORD.

For example, prokinetics might be used to treat patients who also have insulin-dependent diabetes, or infants and children with significantly impaired bowel emptying or severe constipation that doesn't respond to other treatment."

Erythromycin

"This antibiotic, prescribed at low dosages, may improve gastric emptying. Like metoclopramide, erythromycin works by increasing the contractions that move food through the stomach. Food will not remain in the stomach as long as usual, hence there may be less chance of reflux occurring. Possible side effects of erythromycin include nausea, vomiting, and abdominal cramps".

Metoclopramide

"Metoclopramide - brand name Reglan [44], (available in the USA) is a Prokinetic drug that stimulates the muscles of the gastrointestinal tract

---

[44] MedicineNet, Inc., 1996-2014 . *Metoclopramide, Reglan: Drug Facts, Side Effects and Dosing.* [Online]

including the muscles of the lower oesophageal sphincter, stomach, and small intestine by interacting with receptors for acetylcholine and dopamine on gastrointestinal muscles and nerves.

Possible side effects: Reglan can cause serious side effects, including:

- *Abnormal muscle movements called tardive dyskinesia (TD).*
- *These movements happen mostly in the face muscles.*
- *You cannot control these movements.*
- *They may not go away even after stopping Reglan.*
- *There is no treatment for TD*
- *Symptoms may lessen or go away over time after you stop taking Reglan[45]".*

Available at: http://www.medicinenet.com/metoclopramide/article.htm [Accessed 30 June 2014].

[45] Baxter Healthcare Corporation, n.d. *MEDICATION GUIDE REGLAN (Reg-lan) (metoclopramide) injection,* Deerfield, IL 60015 USA: Baxter Healthcare Corporation.

Chapter 10

Food Intolerances

This section is very important as in my research, and experience, I have found that allergies and intolerance to food go hand in hand with reflux. It is important to remember that intolerance and allergies can, and in most cases will, increase the severity of reflux issues.

If your baby has a suspected allergy or intolerance to baby formula or solids, no amount of prescribed medication will bring reflux under control. It is only when the problem food is identified and removed that the symptoms will improve.

What is the difference in allergy V Intolerance?

Food allergies (IgE mediated allergies) can happen when our body's immune systems mistakenly react to a food protein instead of a bacteria or virus. Common food allergies include milk, eggs, wheat, fish and peanuts. However, any food protein can cause a reaction. About 5% of children under the age of 3 are allergic to one or more foods.

While food is one of the most common allergens, medicine, insect bites, latex and exercise can also cause a reaction.

A true food allergy causes an immune system reaction that affects numerous organs and can cause a range of symptoms. In some cases, an allergic reaction to a food can be severe or life-threatening. Anaphylaxis is the most serious type of allergic reaction. It can progress very quickly and may cause death without proper medical intervention.

In contrast, food intolerance symptoms are generally less serious and often limited to digestive problems and can take a while to show a reaction, parents seldom know what foods has caused the reaction as it can be over days even weeks.

Blood tests in babies are said to be inconclusive and may come back clear; however, symptoms or reactions are a strong indication that a baby may not have an allergy but intolerance (Non-IgE mediated allergies). This list is an indication of some of the symptoms your baby/child may present with, not all of them need to be experienced to receive a diagnosis from your medical professional.

Signs & Symptoms of Intolerance

- Watery explosive stool.
- Constipation that can become chronic
- Sneezing
- Wheezing
- Heightened reflux.
- Vomiting
- Itchy, watery eyes
- Eczema like symptoms
- Rash or pimples that resemble baby acne but gradually get worse.
- Red ring around the perennial area of the bum that cream won't clear and can eventually bleed.
- Swollen puffy eyes
- Scratching excessively.
- Generally unwell and cross
- Stomach issues, cramping, bloating.
- Blue vein across the nose, also known as the sugar bug, or Kanmushi in Chinese medicine. When this vein is visible, it is said to be a warning that the child may react to sugar.

- Allergic shiners. These are dark circles under the eyes (bags). This is caused by congestion, which results in swelling of the small blood vessels under the skin.

- Behavioural & Emotional issues,

Our brain and gut communicate with each other on a constant basis. Some professionals believe that the gut and the brain should be regarded as one.

If you have ever experienced the sensation of butterflies or worrying gut wrenching feeling, you may understand this concept better.

When we are emotional or upset or worried we find eating impossible, or some people feel the need to comfort eat when upset.

Our gut is deep rooted with cells of the enteric nervous system (ENS)[46]

Raven experiences Non-IgE mediated allergies and has reactions to a lot of foods. I can tell when she is reacting to certain foods, she gets a red

---

[46]PaddockPhD,Catharine[http://www.medicalnewstoday.com/articles/159914.php] para 5 [Accessed 05 May 2015].

rash around her mouth and her behaviour totally changes. Mango is a huge trigger here for us; in fact, she seems to react badly to most foods that are orange in colour.

The following section is a direct excerpt kindly provided by gikids.org website:

"Frequently asked Questions and answers about Cow's Milk Protein Intolerances (CMPI)[47]

1. What is Cow's Milk Protein Intolerance (CMPI) & What Causes it?

Cow's milk protein intolerance (CMPI) is defined as an abnormal reaction by the body's immune system to protein found in cow's milk. The immune system normally protects our bodies from harm caused by bacteria or viruses.

---

[47] GI for Kids, PLLC, 2003-2014. Paediatric Gastroenterology - Barrett's Esophagus - Diseases - East Tennessee Children's Hospital - GI for Kids, PLLC. [Online] Available at: http://www.giforkids.com/?a=Diseases&b=Barrett%27s%20Esophagus [Accessed 09 June 2014].

In CMPI the immune system reacts unusually to the protein found in cow's milk. This reaction can cause injury in the stomach and intestines.

2. How Common is Cow's Milk Protein Intolerance and Who is at Risk of Developing it?

Risk factors for developing CMPI include having a parent or sibling with atopic or allergic disease (like asthma, eczema, and seasonal allergies). Breastfeeding can in some cases protect infants from developing CMPI.

3. What are the Different Types of Cow's Milk Protein Intolerance?

Cow's milk protein intolerance can be divided into IgE-mediated (immediate reaction) and non-IgE mediated (delayed reaction) types. The two types have different symptoms associated with each.

Immunoglobulin E or IgE is an antibody normally found in humans that causes the symptoms seen with allergies (hives, rashes, wheezing, and runny nose). In IgE-mediated cow's milk protein allergy, symptoms usually start within 2hrs of drinking cow's milk. In non-IgE-mediated CMPI, symptoms happen later, from 48 hours to 1 week after drinking cow's milk.

4. What are the Signs and Symptoms of Cow's Milk Protein Intolerance?

Signs and symptoms of cow's milk protein intolerance are very diverse. The symptoms will usually develop within the first week of starting cow's milk in their diet. Most infants will show signs that involve the skin or the gastrointestinal (GI) system. GI symptoms can include vomiting, abdominal pain, blood in the stools, and diarrhoea. Skin manifestations include hives and eczema. Babies can also present with wheezing, irritability, facial swelling, and poor growth due to poor absorption of nutrients.

5. When Should you Contact or see a Doctor or Paediatric Gastroenterologist?

Red flags: Increased tiredness or lethargy, fevers, severe vomiting or diarrhoea, not tolerating feeding, weight loss, blood in the stools.

6. How is Cow's Milk Protein Intolerance Diagnosed?

Medical history and physical examination are the most helpful in diagnosing CMPI. Describing your child's signs and symptoms (what your child is experiencing) to the physician is very important in making the diagnosis of this disease. The timing of the symptoms in relation to starting feeds with cow's milk protein is also key in diagnosis. Whether there is a family history of allergies, asthma, or eczema can be helpful for diagnosis.

CMPI also is diagnosed after seeing how your child responds to the elimination of cow's milk from the diet.

7. What Tests are used in Children to Diagnose Cow's Milk Protein Intolerance?

Checking for blood in the stool of infants suspected of having CMPI can be helpful in diagnosing this disorder. Blood tests and other invasive studies are not always helpful in diagnosing cow's milk protein intolerance. Your physician may recommend tests to exclude other problems.

8. What is the Treatment for Cow's Milk Protein Intolerance?

The treatment of CMPI includes eliminating cow's milk protein from the infant's diet. Elimination diets are usually started with extensively hydrolysed formulas. These formulas are made up of broken down proteins and are able to be digested without an immune reaction. These formulas will work in 90% of patients with CMPI. In some patients, it is necessary to use amino-acid based formulas, which are formulas containing the individual building blocks of proteins.

In breastfed infants with CMPI, the mother must exclude all dairy and soy products from her diet if she continues to breastfeed. This may be difficult, and is helped by having a dietician discuss hidden sources of dairy and soy with the mother prior to starting the elimination diet.

Giving infant's goat's milk or sheep's milk will not improve CMPI. Soy milk also is not recommended. Many infants will have similar allergic reactions to the proteins in these milks or soy-based formula.

9. What can I Expect if my Child has Cow's Milk Protein Intolerance?

Fortunately, cow's milk protein allergy resolves in 90% of children by the age of 6 years. 50% of infants will have tolerance at age 1 year, and more than 75% will have resolution by 3 years of age.

Most infants that are started on cow's milk-free formulas or breastfed by a mother on a cow's milk-free diet will need to remain on the diet for about 6-12 months. At that point, the child can be challenged with cow's milk, and if they have no reactions, milk can be put back into the child's diet.

10. Where Can I Find Support for my Child and Family?

CMPA Support[48], Jolene Beaton. Listed in Useful websites in the back of the book

---

[48] Jolene Beatson, S. W., n.d. *CMPA Support.* [Online] Available at: http://cowsmilkproteinallergysupport.webs.com/ [Accessed 17 June 2014].

Lactose Intolerance[49]

"Despite the apparent similarity to milk protein allergy above, these are in fact completely different issues. Lactose is a sugar contained in all types of milk. The lactose intolerant baby is unable to produce sufficient quantities of the enzyme lactase required to break down and digest this sugar properly. Instead, bacteria in the gut feast on undigested lactose causing excess quantities of gas, bloating and even diarrhoea. Feeding a baby with lactose free formula can help greatly.

Food Allergy & Breast Feeding

Some studies suggest that if breastfeeding, a mother's diet may affect her baby. Specific foods contain trace elements that can be passed to the baby through breast milk which, so the theory goes, create reactions in baby's gut leading to colic. Foods in mom's diet that have been linked to gassiness in baby include; cow's milk, cruciferous vegetables, beans,

---

[49] Ketomi Distribution, Colic Calm @2013-2014. Colic Calm. [Online] Available at: http://www.coliccalm.com.au/blog/cat/baby-colic-gas-reflux [Accessed 12 April 2014].

peas, acidic foods such as citrus fruits, coffee, strawberries and tomatoes and dairy products, soy and peanuts.

Likewise elements found in formula, such as cow's milk proteins, may affect formula fed babies.

If breastfeeding and your baby show signs of intolerance, discontinue suspected foods in your diet to see if symptoms improve. If this happens, gradually reintroduce specific foods until symptoms return. In this way you can identify the culprit, if indeed food insensitivity is the cause.

Formula fed babies may switch to a hypoallergenic formula" ***(See ref 35)***

Diagnosis/Testing[50]

"To determine if there is a food allergy, a doctor must first find out if the patient is having a harmful (adverse) reaction to a specific food. This includes a patient history and information on what foods are eaten. The next step is to eliminate the food from the diet. If the symptom goes

---

[50] GI for Kids, PLLC, 2003-2014. Paediatric Gastroenterology - Barrett's Esophagus - Diseases - East Tennessee Children's Hospital - GI for Kids, PLLC. [Online] Available at: http://www.giforkids.com/?a=Diseases&b=Barrett%27s%20Esophagus [Accessed 09 June 2014].

away, it may be the food. If the food is eaten again, and the symptom returns, then the food can be confirmed as the cause of the allergic reaction.

A skin prick test can be more realistic in determining a food allergy. Skin tests are rapid, simple, and relatively safe. The skin is pricked with a needle to allow a tiny amount of the suspected food beneath the skin's surface. If a raised bump or reaction develops, it shows an allergy. A positive skin test, along with the history of the allergic reaction to the food eaten, are both considered in the doctor's decision that it is a food allergy.

Patients who have had severe anaphylactic reactions may not be able to have skin tests because it could cause a dangerous reaction. For these patients, blood tests such as the RAST and ELISA can be done to determine the allergy.

The RAST blood test measures the amount of allergen-specific IgE in the blood to detect an allergy to a particular substance. Each allergen-specific IgE antibody test is separate and very specific – such as testing the egg white and then testing the egg yolk. If allergen-specific antibodies are found, allergies are suspected. Having IgE antibodies may only mean that you are sensitized to the allergen. You were exposed, but you may not be allergic. The RAST test should be compared to your history of allergies.

FPIES[51]

The following section with answers to Frequently Asked Questions about FPIES is a direct excerpt from KIDS WITH FOOD ALLERGIES (subsequently abbreviated to KWFA) .

"What Does FPIES Stand For?

FPIES is Food Protein-Induced Enterocolitis Syndrome. It is commonly pronounced "F-Pies", as in "apple pies", though some physicians may refer to it as FIES (pronounced "fees", considering food-protein as one word). Enterocolitis is inflammation involving both the small intestine and the colon (large intestine).

---

[51] Kids with Food Allergies, Inc., 2005-2011. *FPIES: Food Protein Induced entero-colitis Syndrome.* [Online] Available at: http://www.kidswithfoodallergies.org/resourcespre.php?id=99# [Accessed 17 June 2014].

What is FPIES

FPIES is a non-IgE mediated immune reaction in the gastrointestinal system to one or more specific foods, commonly characterised by profuse vomiting and diarrhoea. FPIES is presumed to be cell mediated. Poor growth may occur with continual ingestion. Upon removing the problem food(s), all FPIES symptoms subside.

Note:

Having FPIES does not preclude one from having other allergies/intolerances with the food. The most common FPIES triggers are cow's milk (dairy) and soy. However, any food can cause an FPIES reaction, even those not commonly considered allergens, such as rice, oat and barley.

Children with FPIES may experience what appears to be a severe stomach bug, but the "bug" only starts a couple of hours after the offending food is given. Many FPIES parents have rushed their children to the ER, limp from extreme, repeated projectile vomiting, only to be told, "It's the stomach flu." However, the next time they feed their children the same solids, the dramatic symptoms return.

What Does IgE vs. Cell Mediated hypersensitivity (my parenthesis) mean?

IgE stands for Immunoglobulin E. It is a type of antibody, formed to protect the body from infection that functions in allergic reactions. IgE-mediated reactions are considered immediate hypersensitivity immune system reactions, while Cell mediated reactions are considered delayed hypersensitivity. Antibodies are not involved in cell mediated reactions. For the purpose of understanding FPIES, you can disregard all you know about IgE-mediated reactions.

When Do FPIES Reactions Occur?

FPIES reactions often show up in the first weeks or months of life, or at an older age for the exclusively breastfed child. Reactions usually occur upon introducing first solid foods, such as infant cereals or formulas, which are typically made with dairy or soy. (Infant formulas are considered solids for FPIES purposes.) While a child may have allergies and intolerances to food proteins they are exposed to through breast milk, FPIES reactions usually don't occur from breast milk, regardless of the mother's diet. An FPIES reaction typically takes place when the child has directly ingested the trigger food(s).

What is a Typical FPIES Reaction?

As with all things, each child is different, and the range, severity and duration of symptoms may vary from reaction to reaction. Unlike traditional IgE-mediated allergies, FPIES reactions do not manifest with itching, hives, swelling, coughing or wheezing, etc. Symptoms typically only involve the gastrointestinal system, and other body organs are not involved. FPIES reactions almost always begin with delayed onset vomiting (usually two hours after ingestion, sometimes as late as eight hours after). Symptoms can range from mild (an increase in reflux and several days of runny stools) to life threatening (shock). In severe cases, after repeatedly vomiting, children often begin vomiting bile. Commonly, diarrhoea follows and can last up to several days. In the worst reactions (about 20% of the time), the child has such severe vomiting and diarrhoea that s/he rapidly becomes seriously dehydrated and may go into shock.

What is Shock and what are the Symptoms?

Shock is a life-threatening condition. Shock may develop as the result of sudden illness, injury, or bleeding. When the body cannot get enough blood to the vital organs, it goes into shock

Signs of shock include:

- *Weakness, dizziness, and fainting.*
- *Cool, pale, clammy skin*
- *Weak, fast pulse.*
- *Shallow, fast breathing.*
- *Low blood pressure.*
- *Extreme thirst, nausea, or vomiting*
- *Confusion or anxiety*

How Do You Treat an FPIES Reaction?

Always follow your doctor's emergency plan pertaining to your specific situation. Rapid dehydration and shock are medical emergencies. If your child is experiencing symptoms of FPIES or shock, immediately contact your local emergency services.

If you are uncertain that your child is in need of emergency services, contact 9-1-1* or your physician for guidance.

The most critical treatment during an FPIES reaction is intravenous (IV) fluids, because of the risk and prevalence of dehydration. Children experiencing more severe symptoms may also need steroids and in-hospital monitoring. Mild reactions may be able to be treated at home with oral electrolyte re-hydration (e.g., Pedialyte) (Dioralyte)

Author's Note: The emergency phone number (9-1-1) given in the KWFA text is only available in the USA. In Ireland and the UK the emergency services number is 999. Please check within your own country.

Does FPIES Require Epinephrine (Adrenaline)

Not usually, because adrenaline (epinephrine) reverses IgE-mediated symptoms and FPIES is not IgE-mediated. Based on the patient's history, some doctors might prescribe Epinephrine to reverse specific symptoms of shock (e.g., low blood pressure). However, this is only prescribed in specific cases.

What are Some Common FPIES Triggers?

The most common FPIES triggers are traditional first foods, such as dairy and soy. Other common triggers are rice, oat, barley, green beans, peas, sweet potatoes, squash, chicken and turkey. A reaction to one common food does not mean that all of the common foods will be an issue, but patients are often advised to proceed with caution with those foods. Note that while the above foods are the most prevalent, they are not exclusive triggers. Any food has the potential to trigger an FPIES reaction. Even trace amounts can cause a reaction.

How is FPIES Diagnosed?

FPIES is difficult to diagnose, unless the reaction has happened more than once, as it is diagnosed by symptom presentation. Typically foods that trigger FPIES reactions are negative with standard skin and blood allergy tests (SPT, RAST) because they look for IgE-mediated responses. However as stated before, FPIES is not IgE-mediated.

Atrophy patch testing (APT) is being studied for its effectiveness in diagnosing FPIES, as well as predicting if the problem food is no longer a trigger. Thus, the outcome of APT may determine if the child is a potential candidate for an oral food challenge (OFC). APT involves placing the trigger food in a metal cap, which is left on the skin for 48 hours. The skin is then watched for symptoms in the following days after removal. Please consult your child's doctor to discuss if APT is indicated in your situation.

How Do You Care for a Child With FPIES?

Treatment varies, depending on the patient and his/her specific reactions. Often, infants who have reacted to both dairy and soy formulas will be placed on hypoallergenic or elemental formula. Some children do well breastfeeding. Other children who have fewer triggers may just strictly avoid the offending food(s). New foods are usually introduced very slowly, one food at a time, for an extended period of time per food. Some doctors recommend trialling a single food for up to three weeks before introducing another.

Because it's a rare, but serious condition, in the event of an emergency, it is vital to get the correct treatment. Some doctors provide their patients with a letter containing a brief description of FPIES and its proper treatment. In the event of a reaction, this letter can be taken to the ER with the child.

Is FPIES A Lifelong Condition?

Typically, no it is not. Many children outgrow FPIES by about age three. Note, however, that the time varies per individual and the offending food, so statistics are a guide, but not an absolute. In one study, 100% of children with FPIES reactions to barley had outgrown and were tolerating barley by age three. However, only 40% of those with FPIES to rice, and 60% to dairy tolerated it by the same age.

How Do I know If My Child Has Outgrown FPIES?

Together with your child's doctor, you should determine if/when it is likely that your child may have outgrown any triggers. Obviously, determining if a child has outgrown a trigger is something that needs to be evaluated on a food-by-food basis. As stated earlier, APT testing may be an option to assess oral challenge readiness. Another factor for you and your doctor to consider is if your child would physically be able to handle a possible failed challenge.

When the time comes to orally challenge an FPIES trigger, most doctors familiar with FPIES will want to schedule an in-office food challenge. Some doctors (especially those not practicing in a hospital clinic setting) may choose to challenge in the hospital, with an IV already in place, in case of emergency. Each doctor may have his or her own protocol, but an FPIES trigger is something you should definitely NOT challenge without discussing thoroughly with your doctor.

Be aware that if a child passes the in-office portion of the challenge, it does not mean this food is automatically guaranteed "safe." If a child's delay in reaction is fairly short, a child may fail an FPIES food challenge while still at the office/hospital. For those with longer reaction times, it may not be until later that day that symptoms manifest. Some may react up to three days later. Delay times may vary by food as well. If a child has FPIES to multiple foods, one food may trigger symptoms within four hours. A different food may not trigger symptoms until six or eight hours after ingestion.

How is FPIES Different from MPIES, MSPIES, MSPI, Etc.?

MPIES (Milk-Protein induced Enterocolitis syndrome) is FPIES to cow's milk only.

MSPIES (Milk and Soy-protein induced Enterocolitis syndrome) is FPIES to milk and soy. Some doctors do create these subdivisions, while others declare that milk and soy are simply the two most common FPIES triggers and give the diagnosis of "FPIES to milk and/or soy".

MSPI is milk and soy protein intolerance. Symptoms are those of allergic colitis and can include colic, vomiting, diarrhoea and blood in stools. These reactions are not as severe or immediate as an FPIES reaction.

Parent's Experience

"I first realised something else was wrong when his reflux got worse instead of better with weaning. Eating made him miserable.

He would scream, thrash and refuse to sleep. It was only when we switched to a hypoallergenic formula and cut out all food that things improved. Then I realised my hunch was right. Food was driving his reflux; not the other way around as his doctors believed. His diet is very limited still but he's a happy toddler and no longer a screaming baby".

"My instincts told me right from the start that my baby was suffering with more than just reflux. Every single formula he tried was problematic including all the amino acid based ones (which were more troublesome than the other formulas).

We tried weaning at around 18 weeks on doctor's advice and each food we tried gave the same reaction - heightened reflux and spit up, facial marking and swelling, disturbed sleeping patterns, wind and tummy ache as well as either diarrhoea or constipation. It took a huge amount of convincing for doctors to believe us that this was happening but we kept fighting until they listened. It wasn't until our son had an acute FPIES reaction that everything fell into place and he got a diagnosis. The other reactions he was experiencing are known as chronic FPIES reactions and much harder to make a diagnosis as each child has different symptoms whereas an acute FPIES reaction is fairly textbook. At 14 months of age - we still only have one safe food but we are hopeful that things will improve the older he gets.

The lack of knowledge of this condition and how to manage it is frustrating and has left us feel like we have been very much left to our own devices to deal with it and get on with it. With each food trial, there are repercussions from reactions - some more severe than others. But we have no other choice but to plough on and keep going to try and get some variation for our son's diet."

Extract from Monica Brogans online Blog: Gut Allergy Mummy

"I became a mum for the first time in August 2013 to an adorable baby boy called Caolán. From get up go we had issues around feeding with undiagnosed severe posterior and anterior tongue ties, cow's milk protein intolerance and horrendous acid reflux. At ten weeks old, my baby was admitted to hospital with a viral infection known as bronchitis. Caolán was treated with antibiotics for this infection and from here on in, our situation went from bad to worse. It spiralled into something that became the start of a very long journey, which has taken us to where we are today.

We were passed from one health care professional to the next and sadly, our concerns and suggestions about his condition were constantly dismissed and shrugged off as we were "first time parents".

Caolán had several hospital admissions after that initial admission at 10 weeks and his reflux was always completely uncontrolled despite being on a high dose of medication to try and treat it. I couldn't leave the house with him, he was so bad – he would scream and cry and draw much unwanted attention from other people as they sat and watched, casting judgement on my parental skills and in their eyes, the inability to control my baby.

They had no idea of what we had to endure on a daily basis and how much pain our baby was in. It was just so much easier to stay at home, especially when Caolán started to become mobile as we could not risk him accidentally ingesting something he shouldn't, in case it would trigger a reaction.

It took 15 months for us to finally get an official diagnosis and the right medical treatment for Caolán. This only happened when we took matters into our own hands and found help from world leading field experts in gut related allergies based across the water in Great Ormond Street Hospital, London.

Our first encounter was with an amazingly knowledgeable dietician who specialises in this area. She confirmed everything we had suspected and researched ourselves based on the symptoms Caolán was presenting with. She felt there was most definitely some kind of EGID condition present, called FPIES a very inflamed gut and a secondary fructose malabsorption condition. She also felt that he was possibly suffering with delayed gastric emptying of the gut/gut dysmotility so she put together a plan in terms of food trials and referred us on to her colleague who is a paediatric gastroenterologist and a world leading expert in his field, for further investigation.

In our opinion, we just got Caolán to him in time. In the run up to our consultation with him – Caolán had endured a number of food fails coupled with a few viral infections and his gut was in a very, very bad way. He had lost complete tolerance to his one and only safe food (oats) and was barely tolerating his formula. He was in a terrible way symptomatically. I was also 32 weeks pregnant with our second baby so we were anxious to try and get some control on the matter before our next baby arrived. We travelled to London to meet our new paediatrician and just

163

minutes into our consultation with him – relief started to flood over me. We finally found someone who listened, explained and most importantly of all, he believed every single word I said about what had been going on with Caolán's symptoms to date.

He did not question a single thing and instead he took the time to make us feel at ease and explain what the reasons behind these symptoms were and what was causing Caolán's inability to tolerate any food to date. He felt the antibiotics administered at 10 weeks of age completely destroyed the lining of an already very sensitive guy. He described Caolán's stomach as burning inferno – that was currently burning out of control. He said for every food we trailed, it was just like adding petrol to a fire because his little gut was so badly inflamed. He also felt Caolán's physical appearance suggested a very inflamed gut. The tone of his skin, swelling around his eyes and his bum was red.

He then proceeded to prescribe medication; immediately we were to administer an aggressive dose of steroids over a ten day period, he wanted us to continue on giving him Ketotifen (an antihistamine) that he had been on since 7 months of age and he prescribed nalcrom (an anti-allergy drug) 3 times a day. In addition – he told us to stop losec completely as it was just a waste of time for him to be taking it when it wasn't controlling the reflux.

He then scheduled scopes for 4 weeks later for further investigation and biopsies. Caolán was diagnosed with FPIES, severe non-IgE allergies and severe gut inflammation. We got more help and support in 30 mins with our new paediatrician than what we had in 15 months in Ireland. We were so elated that we had found much needed help and we finally had a treatment plan for our beloved little boy.

We noticed a difference almost immediately on the new meds. His symptoms slowly but surely started to subside. By the fourth week (week of scopes) he really was a different child. The results of the scope that came back were positive as the new medication had started to work. The scopes showed the inflammation was all in his bowel and intestine. Our Paediatrician felt that it was the inflammation in his bowel that had been driving the reflux. Even though losec had been unable to keep the reflux under control, it had thankfully managed to prevent any damage to his upper GI Tract from the continuous acid burning he would of been experiencing with the uncontrolled reflux.

Biopsies from his bowel and intestine showed evidential signs of inflammation that were now both in recovery. His lymph nodes were still very swollen and inflamed and other findings included marked lymphonodular hyperplasia, which is a very, very rare find, but from what we are told, associated with a child with severe allergies. Thankfully, all other results and findings came back ok. But he was elemental at the time of scopes and not reacting. After these results, our Ped felt we were in a good place and Caolán's gut was now stable enough to recommence food trials.

He feels our long term prognosis is good because we got medical intervention when we did and is very hopeful that Caolán will outgrow these conditions between 5-7 years old. We are just so lucky we did not give up our fight in trying to get him diagnosed – despite being told many times along the way that it was "just reflux" and he would grow out of these food allergies and reactions by the age of one! Because of our persistency – we have saved our son from any real long term damage. As well as all of this, we now have answers and more importantly, a diagnosis that comes with an action plan to treat his condition. We have something to work towards and there is light at the end of the tunnel.

In the meantime, we have to try and keep positive, soldier on with food trials and deal with each reaction, taking each day as it comes. It is so important to keep Caolán "safe" from accidental exposure to trigger foods and put our best foot forward as we continue on this journey of the unknown.

He has huge issues with corn and is extremely sensitive to products derived from corn. Unfortunately for us – this is a really big problem as corn can be found in so many things; household cleaning products, shampoo, bath lotion, soap, toilet paper, kitchen roll, hardback books, sun cream to name but a few. These products can often result in accidental exposure and trigger a reaction.

Our second baby was born in January 2015 and again, we had feeding issues from birth. Our little boy Oisín spent nearly the first four weeks of his life in the neonatal unit at our local hospital. We were able to act much faster this time around as we are now well seasoned allergy parents! We knew all the marker signs straight off.

Our babies look totally healthy and like any normal child on the outside, but appearances can be seriously deceptive. Food could have lethal consequences for our oldest boy Caolán as. FPIES is a non-IgE allergy and the most severe type of a reaction in the non-IgE allergy spectrum. It can have fatal consequences. FPIES can be compared in severity to a serious anaphylactic shock in the IgE allergy spectrum. It is a very frightening experience but thankfully most children tend to also outgrow this condition by the age of approximately 4.

Caolán's FPIES condition along with his diagnosis of severe multiple non-IgE allergies, makes day to day living extremely complicated in our home. It is a constant battle of food trials and reactions with bouts of normal childhood illnesses and teething all thrown into the mix for good measure!

The hardest part of this is that with non-IgE allergies – there are no tests to determine what food can cause an allergic reaction. The only way of finding out what foods are and not safe, is by carrying out food trials for every single food and ingredient that you wish to feed your child. It means that when we do start to get some "safe" foods – everything he eats will have to be pre- pared and cooked by me and I will have to become extremely creative in making food seem interesting and appealing, serving it in different ways and learn how to substitute ingredients in a recipe for ingredients that he can have.

Life at present is all about keeping our babies safe from harm and any foods or products that they could potentially react to. Obviously Oisín is much too young for any kind of food consumption other than formula at present. But we still need to ensure that in the likelihood he is as reactive as his big brother Caolán that cross contamination of food of any sort does not occur until we are ready to start weaning and trailing''.

Further Reading and information about allergy can be found on Monica's Blog   http://gutallergymummy.com/

Chapter 11

Faecal Calprotectin

A Screening Test for Detecting Gastrointestinal Inflammation in Children

By listening to feedback from members of the SRI support group, I have been become aware that Faecal Calprotecin testing[52] is now recommended more and more in cases where inflammation is suspected in presented cases of gastroenteritis.

Studies are underway in Ireland and the UK to assess both its cost-effectiveness as a diagnostic test and well as its potential as an alternative to the more invasive procedures of surgical endoscopy.

---

[52] Info available online. Available at
http://labtestsonline.org/understanding/analytes/calprotectin/tab/test. Accessed Mar 2015

Although relatively new and not yet widely used, both countries seem to have a positive view on calprotectin testing based on the aforementioned criteria; cost and diagnostic usefulness.

Ireland has a *National Centre for Paediatric Gastroenterology, Hepatology and Nutrition* for paediatric gastroenterology and the Faecal Calprotectin test is now being conducted in Our lady's Children's Hospital in Crumlin in Dublin where the Irish studies are being undertaken. The following paragraphs contain general information about calprotectin and explain the background for the calprotectin test.

What is Calprotectin?

Calprotectin is a protein found in the intestine during periods of inflammation. Intestinal inflammation can be the result of a wide range of underlying problems such as a bacterial infection, some parasitic infections, colorectal cancer, Irritable Bowel Disease (IBD) or Crohn's Disease, to name a few. The symptoms of these potentially serious illnesses listed above may be very similar to those observed in cases of non-inflammatory conditions such as Irritable Bowel Syndrome (IBS).

The range and severity of symptoms can vary from one person to the next as well as over time. Symptoms may include one or more of the following:

- Bloody or watery diarrhoea
- Abdominal cramps or pain
- Fever
- Weight loss
- Rectal bleeding
- Weakness

Unfortunately, the symptoms of IBD and IBS are so similar that people with less serious IBS may be subjected to unnecessary, uncomfortable and invasive surgical procedures such as endoscopy (colonoscopy or sigmoidoscopy) to examine the intestines. These internal examinations are often coupled to a small tissue biopsy to evaluate the levels of inflammation and monitor any changes in tissue structures.

Testing for calprotectin can help doctors distinguish between these non-inflammatory conditions and IBD, since calprotectin isn't usually present in the intestines of an individual with a non-inflammatory bowel disorder.

Although the incidence of childhood IBD seems to be increasing, early[53] results in national statistics in Ireland suggest that up to 70% of children referred for paediatric gastroenterology screening do not have IBD.

When is it Ordered?

A Faecal Calprotectin test may be ordered when a person presents with symptoms (listed above) suggestive of gastrointestinal inflammation and a doctor wants to distinguish between IBD and a non-inflammatory bowel condition.

Calprotectin testing, therefore, adds to the diagnostic toolbox, since it helps to guide doctors in identifying the underlying cause for the symptoms presented. Based on the results of a calprotectin test, a decision about whether more invasive procedures (endoscopy etc.) are required or not can be made.

When a person has already been diagnosed with IBD, a calprotectin test may be ordered whenever a relapse is suspected, both to confirm disease activity and to evaluate its severity.

---

[53] Trends in Hospitalizations of Children With Inflammatory Bowel Disease Within the United States From 2000 to 2009. Journal of Investigative Medicine, 2013 DOI:10.231/JIM.0b013e31829a4e25

The Faecal Calprotectin Test – What is it and How it is Performed?

Calprotectin is measured in stool samples (faeces). Calprotectin is present in the blood, urine and stools of all people, including healthy people. However, the levels of calprotectin in the faeces can rise dramatically when an inflammatory bowel condition is present. Elevated stool calprotectin levels are indicative of the migration (movement) of neutrophils (a type of white blood cell) to the intestinal walls, an event which occurs during intestinal inflammation.

As faecal calprotectin levels are tested against a "cut off" level (x mg calprotectin/g faeces), calprotectin levels are determined to be negative (below cut off) or elevated (above cut off) or severely high (highly elevated above cut off). The results of a calprotectin test are normally given as:

The amount of calprotectin (milligram/mg) per gram (g) of faeces

Faecal calprotectin testing can also be used to monitor the activity and severity of these inflammatory diseases.

What Does the Test Result Mean?

A low calprotectin result suggests that symptoms observed are likely due to a non-inflammatory bowel disorder or a viral gastrointestinal infection. People with low calprotectin results often don't require a confirmatory endoscopy.

Moderately elevated calprotectin levels may indicate that there is some inflammation or that the person's condition is worsening. A second test revealing moderately elevated or further elevated calprotectin levels is likely to prompt further investigation and this may involve a confirmatory endoscopic examination. When calprotectin levels are considered to be high doctors are likely to order a colonoscopy or sigmoidoscopy as a follow-up to determine the cause of inflammation, taking into account all symptoms observed. Faecal calprotectin levels are often very high in people who have recently been diagnosed with IBD.

Related Tests

Additional tests may be ordered in conjunction with faecal calprotectin testing in order to make the most accurate diagnosis possible. Such tests can include:

> ➤ A stool culture to detect a bacterial infection. This is where a sample of your stool will be check in the lab for the growth of disease-causing bacteria. This test typically takes a few days.

> ➤ A stool white blood cell test. The presence of leukocytes (a certain type of white blood cells) in the stool is indicative of bacterial infections and/or inflammatory bowel conditions such as Crohn's disease.

> ➤ And/or a faecal occult blood test (FOBT). This test is used to detect the presence of tiny amounts of blood in stool samples that may not be seen with the naked eye.

If a doctor suspects inflammation, blood tests that detect inflammation in the body may be ordered, such as tests to measure:

> ➤ Erythrocyte sedimentation rate (ESR)
> ➤ And/or C-reactive protein (CRP)

These blood tests can ascertain whether or not there is inflammation in the body but they cannot identify the location of this inflammation. This means that additional blood and stool testing may be performed depending on the specific set of symptoms and the suspected underlying cause.

The calprotectin test is related to the lactoferrin stool test. Like calprotectin, lactoferrin is released by white blood cells in the stool and is associated with intestinal inflammation. Of these two tests, calprotectin seems to have been the most extensively studied, and it seems to be ordered more frequently than lactoferrin.

An elevated calprotectin indicates that inflammation is likely present in the gastrointestinal tract but does not indicate exactly where or the cause. In general, the degree of elevation is associated with the severity of the inflammation.

Is There Anything Else I Should Know

It is worthwhile noting that an increase in faecal calprotectin can arise as a result of anything which leads to bowel inflammation. It doesn't always mean disease per se. For instance, faecal calprotectin levels may be increased following intestinal tissue damage and bleeding that is sometimes seen during extended period of use/overuse use of non-steroidal anti-inflammatory drugs (NSAIDS) such as aspirin and ibuprofen.

Occasionally, calprotectin levels may be low, even though inflammation is present. This is known as a false negative, and is most frequently observed in children. Conversely, false positives may also occur. The usage of PPIs, in particular omeprazole is associated with significantly increased faecal calprotectin levels, so a positive result in a PPI user doesn't necessarily mean that intestinal inflammation is present[54], and should be interpreted with caution. Such a result may be followed up with other tests for intestinal inflammation.

---

[54] Poullis A, Foster R, Mendall MA, Shreeve D, Wiener K (2003). "Proton pump inhibitors are associated with elevation of faecal calprotectin and may affect specificity". Eur J Gastroenterol Hepatol 15(5): 573–4; author reply 574. doi:10.1097/00042737-200305000-00021. PMID 12702920.

Common Questions

1. Can a Blood Test be Substituted For a Stool Calprotectin Test?

In general, no. There are blood tests used to detect inflammation (CRP, ESR), but they do not provide the same information about gastrointestinal inflammation as the stool calprotectin test.

2. What Can I Do to Decrease My Calprotectin?

Since faecal calprotectin levels are an indicator of gastrointestinal inflammation, they are not affected by lifestyle changes. If your faecal calprotectin levels are increased due to an infection, they will most likely return to normal once the infection has passed. If it is due to IBD, then it will rise and fall with disease activity. In the rare case that an elevated faecal calprotectin level is caused by non-steroidal anti inflammatory drug (NSAID) therapy, then it is likely to return to normal when the medication is discontinued.

3. Can the Faecal Calprotectin Test be Performed in My Doctor's Office?

No. The equipment required for this test is laboratory-based and is not offered by all laboratories. A stool sample is likely to be sent to a laboratory for testing and it may take several days before results become available. Your doctor will be able to provide with a more realistic time frame for your Faecal Calprotectin test results.

Chapter 12

Weaning Your Baby onto Solids

When it is time to wean your baby onto solids there are many things you may have to consider.

We felt weaning would be the answers to all our prayers. Many of us are led to believe by medical professionals that weaning a baby with GORD will significantly reduce problems.

This, however, in most cases, is the furthest thing from the truth as many foods can exacerbate and flare symptoms of GORD and cause horrendous pain for the baby. At the start, we only had a few safe foods and we stuck to them for a long time. It is important to remember that every baby is different and it is all trial and error. I'm afraid what works for one will not work for another.

Having a baby with CMSPI is very tough as everything seems to contain dairy, even probiotics. A shopping trip would take me hours while I scoured every label. Also, it is extremely hard for GORD parents to purchase baby food without food triggers in them. I avoided any citrus fruits. I stuck to pear; it was very safe for us. Apple seems to be in almost every fruit product on the market.

Why aren't there reflux friendly solid foods on the market?

When weaning, take it slow. Keep a diary of foods given and watch for changes in behaviour.

If at all possible, make your own food. When Raven was old enough, I used to make a big pot of stew (an Irish dish) on a Saturday and put it into six containers and freeze them. Very handy, cheap and she loved them. More importantly, I knew exactly what she was getting!

Parent's Experiences

"Weaning is a difficult one because every baby is so different and while all advice is great it's definitely trial and error and the error is where the heartache and the reflux flare ups appear. For baby I started on the usual pear, carrot, butternut squash and to thicken them and keep tummy settled and acid at bay I added a

little baby rice to start with. But rice by itself just constipated her. Anything processed flares her reflux so I make everything for her. Only tip would be patience and when others try to shove crap into your little one saying 'oh it will do her no harm', stand strong; they wouldn't be the ones pacing the floor at three am".

"I found that too, the doctors said weaning would improve the reflux but if anything it made it worse. They also told me she would grow out if it at 3 months to 6 but she never did she's 2 now and still on Losec".

"For us I found the main thing was waiting until she was some way settled. We didn't start weaning until she was six months and started on baby rice, carrot, sweet potato etc. all the usual's. She was still pretty unsettled then though so it's really only in the last few months - probably since she turned one - which we can tell what doesn't agree with her. Gluten is still a no, beef is a no, no cow's milk but regular formula and cheese and yogurts are ok. Gluten free muffins I made her are fine but gluten free banana bread with virtually the same ingredients (but a bit more maple syrup and butter) drove her cracked up all night scratching and hiccupping and screaming. Spinach drove her mad too last time I tried it though we had thought she was ok with it so who knows".

"A lot of PHNs and GPs who are not specialists in childhood reflux are still following outdated advice to wean early when all the specialist evidence indicates this is actually harmful to their sensitive systems. Do not wean before 6 months in most cases as you are doing more harm than good. I recently heard of someone advised to give a 3 month old baby rice & flat 7up. That child may be paying for this for the rest of his life with stomach issues. They are so fragile".

"Another important thing to remember is that the new advice re allergies is that waiting to introduce foods such as dairy or wheat has little benefit, they are either going to have issues or they aren't. Gluten should be introduced extremely slowly after 6 months but before 7 months".

"I don't think it cures reflux if a baby has true reflux (vomiting reflux), it seems to work better with Silent Reflux just from speaking with other mums. With my daughter's reflux it was purely anatomical i.e. her oesophagus needed to strengthen and no medication or different formula was going to do that. The week she learned to sit unaided at 7 months her reflux disappeared. She had had severe puking of every feed from birth to the point that I truly believed it would never end.

I know a lot still battle past this age but it is true that for a large portion this strengthening of muscles does seem to fix things between 7-12 months of age. Beyond that you are possibly looking at dairy intolerances or other stomach issues but I'm not a doctor. I have only ever dealt with pure classic reflux. I've been there and unable to leave the house. It is horrendous but in our case and a lot of cases they do recover and I wouldn't mess with weaning early and risk complications with that".

Chapter 13

GORD Common Cause of Ear, Nose & Throat Problems

GORD can cause a multitude of other medical problems. When Raven turned 12 months her symptoms flared, she had a throat infection which turned into tonsillitis, acute tonsillitis. She had a chest infection, bronchitis and was on steroids and inhalers. She then had a burst eardrum from frequent infections that caused her ear to bleed. We met a doctor in A&E in Our Lady's Hospital, Crumlin, that told us the acid was causing the good bacteria at the back of the throat to deplete, thus causing infection. She also informed us that aspirations of food into the lungs will cause issues that antibiotics will not clear up and she recommended we put Raven back on a PPI. We did this and she has not had issues since I really hope I don't jinx myself now! Reflux mothers always say this!

I found some brilliant information from the archives of *MARCI-Kids*. If you are finding your baby has serious problem issues with his/her ear, nose and/or throat, GORD could be the cause of or could contribute to these health issues.

The following sections are direct excerpts from the archives of *MARCI-Kids:*[55]

Introduction

Intermittent reflux of stomach contents into the esophagus is a normal physiological process. It occurs because of transient relaxation of the sphincter located where the esophagus connects to the stomach. Gastroesophageal reflux is considered to be abnormal or pathologic if it produces symptoms, and is then referred to as gastroesophageal reflux disease (GERD).

GERD is a well-documented and common occurrence among adults, but during the last twenty years, it has been increasingly

---

[55] MARCI-Kids.com, 2007. EXTRA ESOPHAGEAL REFLUX AND SYMPTOMS OF THE EAR, NOSE, THROAT. [Online] Available at http://web.archive.org/web/20081012221121/http://www.marci-kids.com/eerintro.html [Accessed 21 May 2014].

recognized as a clinical entity among children and infants. GERD most commonly results in vomiting, abdominal or chest pain, heartburn, arousal from sleep, and regurgitation (spitting up).

*If gastric reflux reaches the level of the pharynx (throat) by moving past both the lower and upper oesophageal sphincter it is termed extra-oesophageal reflux (EER). Evidence is accumulating that EER can be a factor in disorders of the upper and lower airway in both adults and children (reviewed in **1, 2**).*

*Infants may be especially predisposed to reflux-related problems because they have relatively more reflux events than adults. In a survey of 948 infants, it was found that nearly 50% of babies less than 3 months old had reflux events that resulted in regurgitation or spitting up at least once a day **(3)**. The number increased to a maximum of 67% of 4-month-olds. By 1 year of age, percent of infants with daily regurgitation events was less than 5%.*

Although symptoms of GERD are fairly easy to diagnose, extra-oesophageal reflux is a more difficult diagnosis. "Silent reflux" or atypical reflux in which the patient has no gastrointestinal symptoms is very common in children with upper and lower airway complaints. Determining the involvement of

EER requires verifying its presence by some diagnostic methodology.

A methodology commonly used to determine whether a person has gastroesophageal reflux is to measure acidity by means of a pH-detecting "probe" placed at the lower esophageal sphincter (LES). However, traditional pH probes placed to detect acid reflux at the LES can easily overlook EER in the child. A significant percentage of children who have EER show normal pH data from probes placed at the LES (4, 5). Therefore, a better approach to EER diagnosis is to monitor pH in the pharynx or upper esophagus. Although pharyngeal probes provide excellent measures of EER, they are uncomfortable for some children because the procedure involves insertion of rubber tubing through the nose. Parents also shy away, especially once they learn the tubing must stay in the nose for 24 hours.

An innovative alternative for diagnosing EER is the Bravo pH capsule. This capsule is wireless, and is placed in the upper esophagus just behind the upper esophageal sphincter (6). The Bravo system has been a very good way to measure upper esophageal reflux without any tubing.

In this chapter we focus on how EER results in damage to cells and tissues of the larynx and upper respiratory tract. We also discuss a number of ear, nose, throat, and laryngeal disorders commonly encountered in paediatric patients and examine evidence for the role of EER in causing or exacerbating these conditions.

How Reflux Affects the Airway

The larynx, or voice box, acts as a two-way valve to prevent aspiration of food and liquids into the lungs during swallowing. During breathing, the larynx is open, allowing air to move in and out of the lungs via the trachea, but during swallowing, the larynx closes off the airway.

Even so, the proximity of the airway to the esophageal entrance makes the potential for reflux to enter the airway very high in certain situations. When a person is lying flat, refluxing gastric contents can readily flow into the esophagus to the level of the larynx and throat. Babies are especially prone to EER because their lower esophageal sphincter doesn't reach maturity until 18 months and therefore doesn't always function fully to keep gastric contents in the stomach.

Acid and the digestive enzyme pepsin are responsible for the damaging effects of reflux. Stomach tissue is most protected against their damaging effects, but even so, erosions and ulcers can develop. While not nearly as resistant to the effects of acid and pepsin as the stomach tissue, the esophagus is adapted to handle some acid exposure that occurs due to intermittent physiological reflux. Peristalsis, which is rhythmic, wavelike movement of the esophagus, helps push reflux back into the stomach. The esophagus secretes mucus that forms a protective barrier against the corrosive effects of the reflux. The esophagus is also lined by a specialized layer of cells called stratified squamous epithelium that secretes bicarbonate ions, which can neutralize the acid. Even these protective mechanisms in place, acid may still penetrate the epithelial layers and irritate nerve endings, which results in the sensation of "heartburn."

Unlike the stomach and esophagus, the respiratory tract is extremely sensitive to the damaging effects of gastric fluids. The respiratory tract is lined by a cell layer called pseudo-stratified, ciliated columnar epithelium, which is very different in structure from the epithelium in the esophagus. Respiratory epithelia *possess tiny hairs called cilia that perform a protective function. The sweeping action of the cilia keeps the airway clear by removing mucus from the respiratory tract. The cilia also help eliminate infectious and allergenic materials from the body because any bacteria, viruses, dust, pollen or mold that float onto the cilia also are swept out of the airway.*

When repeatedly exposed to reflux, the respiratory columnar epithelium sometimes will change into stratified squamous epithelium like that found in the oesophagus. Although more resistant to the damaging effects of reflux, squamous cells do not possess cilia. By causing the loss of cilia, EER compromises an essential cleansing process in the respiratory tract.

Sometimes when explaining to patients the difference between the ability of the oesophagus and the airway to tolerate reflux, we use the analogy of the oesophagus being a rubber hose and the airway being tissue paper. While not entirely accurate, it does paint a picture of the relative sensitivities of the two.

Although direct irritation of the respiratory tract by acid and pepsin can bring about the signs and symptoms of airway disease, reflux can also have an indirect, or referred, effect on the airway even if it never leaves the oesophagus. This indirect effect comes about because the oesophagus and airway are connected to a common central nerve called the vagus.

When acid refluxing into the lower oesophagus interacts with special structures called receptors, nerve impulses can arc backwards along the vagus to cause spastic closure of the larynx (laryngospasm). This reflexive response of the airway to reflux is yet another way in which the body protects itself from aspiration.

Common Ear, Nose and Throat Conditions Resulting from EOR

A number of ear, nose and throat disorders commonly encountered in children and infants have been found to be associated with Extra-Oesophageal Reflux (EOR). For some disorders, the association is likely causative, that is, the acid and pepsin in reflux are directly responsible for the signs and symptoms associated with the condition.

For other disorders, EOR is not necessarily causative, but the presence of reflux can make the signs and symptoms much worse. In a few cases, it has been speculated that worsening of symptoms is because the condition increases the likelihood that reflux can escape the oesophagus and get into the airway. In other words, rather than EOR causing the condition, the condition causes EOR. This section provides an overview of the signs and symptoms of laryngeal and upper airway disorders commonly encountered in paediatric practice and how EOR can bring about or aggravate these disorders. The role of anti-reflux therapy in treating these conditions is also discussed.

Effects of EOR on the Larynx or Voice Box

The larynx is anatomically just in front of the espohagus and therefore is very susceptible to the effects of EOR. Multiple sites of the larynx can be irritated and cause a number of different signs and symptoms. Some of these include: chronic cough, hoarseness with or without vocal cord nodules, laryngeal ulcers, and vocal cord dysfunction.

Cough

Cough is one symptom commonly associated with irritation of the larynx. Cough is a protective reflex that removes irritants or infectious organisms such as those causing pneumonia. Irritants are detected by "cough receptors," which are nerve endings located in the larynx and other parts of the respiratory tree. Receptors are also located in the naso- and oro-pharynx (throat), the sinuses, and the ears (7). Through coughing, the airway tries to relieve itself of its acid load as best it can. However, persistent cough can itself further irritate the airway. EOR is an important agent in chronic cough, that is, coughing that continues for three to eight weeks. Excluding infectious diseases, EOR is the third most common cause of chronic cough in children and the most common cause in infants 0-18 months old (8).

Hoarseness

Hoarseness is another symptom that can be associated with the deleterious effects of reflux on the larynx. Hoarseness is a general term for any abnormal voice quality, but voice quality can be further described as breathy or harsh, husky or rough, strident, or coarse. Though voice intensity varies with the amount of air pressure against vocal cord resistance, voice quality is primarily determined by length, tension, strength of movement, mass, or position of the vocal cords (9). Any aberration of length or tension of the vibrating segment, mass, posture, or strength of the vocal cords may result in hoarseness. In a study of children aged 2-12 years old who had chronic hoarseness for more than six months, 70% of them were found to also have GERD (10).

When researchers directly examined the vocal cords of these children, one child's vocal cords looked normal, but the remainder had a variety of abnormalities that included cord swelling, nodules, and evidence of healing ulcerations.

Paradoxical Vocal Cord Dysfunction (PVCD)

Another abnormality of the vocal cords that can be associated with damage from reflux is paradoxical vocal cord dysfunction (PVCD). During breathing, normally functioning vocal cords should move into an open position to allow free flow of air through the larynx. In PVCD, the vocal cords are inappropriately closed with breathing. When cord movement is not synchronous with breathing, voice quality isn't affected, but it creates a sensation of airway obstruction. PVCD can be quite distressing and mimic asthma or severe aspiratory airway obstruction. In rare cases, it has resulted in the placement of a tracheotomy *tube to assist breathing. PVCD is most commonly found in teenagers **(11)**, but cases masquerading as bilateral vocal cord paralysis have been reported in newborns **(12)**. Reflux therapy resolves PVCD and may be curative **(11, 12)**.*

Stridor and Laryngomalacia

Another sign of a problem in the airway is stridor, which is a coarse, high-pitched sound when breathing in. Stridor results from turbulent, rapid air flow through a narrowed portion of the airway. Because a number of airway disorders can cause stridor, a physician should explore all possibilities when evaluating patients with stridor, but EOR may play a significant role in those conditions most commonly associated with stridor.

*Airway abnormalities present at birth are responsible for 87% of stridor cases in infants **(13)**. The most common of these congenital abnormalities is laryngomalacia. **(13)** Laryngomalacia refers to an abnormal floppiness of the laryngeal tissues just forward of the vocal cords at the airway entrance. Stridor results because upon inspiration, these floppy tissues get pulled into the opening of the airway, narrowing the diameter of the opening by* *partially blocking it. Although aspiratory breathing is noisy, breathing on expiration is normal, as is the voice.*

Parents may notice their baby has noisy breathing at birth, but usually laryngomalacia-associated stridor becomes most noticeable at 1-2 months when the infant is becoming more active and making more demands on the airway. Respiratory effort and noisy breathing typically get worse before they resolve, usually by 18 months of age.

Two studies have shown a strong association between laryngomalacia and gastroesophageal reflux. In one study, 80% of infants with stridor due to laryngomalacia also had gastroesophageal reflux (14). In another, more recent study, the severity of laryngomalacia was shown to be directly related to the severity of gastroesophageal reflux (15).

The co-association of laryngomalacia and reflux may be a common manifestation of neuromuscular immaturity that simultaneously results in flaccid airway structures and poor oesophageal sphincter tone (14), which may explain why symptoms often disappear as the child matures. Another possibility is that EOR is a secondary effect of the laryngomalacia in which the inspiration of air against the narrowed airway creates a suction effect that pulls reflux up and out of the oesophagus (14). Either way, reflux can cause a worsening of symptoms of laryngomalacia because the inflammation and swelling of the laryngeal tissues result in a greater obstruction of the airway. Aggressive reflux therapy is recommended (5).

Croup and Subglottic Stenosis (SGS)

Reflux may also play a role in children who suffer from repeated cases of croup. Symptoms of croup include stridor, a barking cough, hoarseness, and difficulty breathing. In children older than a year, an isolated case of croup often comes on the heels of an upper respiratory infection and is usually due to a virus-induced inflammation of the larynx. However, infants less than one year old who have repeated cases of croup may have a condition called subglottic stenosis (SGS), which is an abnormal narrowing of the sub glottis, a region of the larynx located below the vocal cords. Different severities of SGS exist and are graded 1-4, with a Grade 1 being the least severe and Grade 4 representing nearly complete obstruction of the airway.

Infants can be born with SGS, but they can also develop SGS due to physical injury to the larynx. Physical injury includes damage caused by acid reflux. Studies in animals in which direct application of acid to the larynx resulted in the formation of SGS confirm a causal association between EER and acquired SGS (16). One study has shown that infants who have recurrent cases of severe croup requiring hospitalisation are more likely to have an additional diagnosis of reflux (17), and another reported that 80% of children undergoing surgery to repair their SGS had at least one positive test for EER (18).

A mild, Grade-1 SGS that would normally not be noticed can be exacerbated by EOR or recurrent viral illness. Children with Grade-1 SGS may spontaneously improve as they get older, and often anti-reflux medication is all that is needed to keep the airway sufficiently open until the SGS resolves. Severe SGS requires surgical intervention, but anti-reflux medications help improve the success rate of these surgeries and reduce the need for additional operations, presumably because healing can occur more readily in the absence of acid (19, 20).

Effects of EOR on the Pharynx, Sinuses, & Ears

Not only can EOR irritate the larynx, it can also irritate the pharynx (throat). Reflux can flow up into the oro- and

200

naso-pharynx and may even reach the nasal and sinus cavities. EOR has accordingly been implicated in a number of symptoms and disorders of the pharynx, nose, sinuses, and ears. Pharyngeal signs and symptoms associated with or caused by EOR include: sensations of choking or a lump in the throat with or without constant throat clearing, adenoid enlargement, rhino sinusitis, and Eustachian tube dysfunction and middle ear infections.

Globus Pharyngeus (Lump in the Throat)

Inflammation of the pharynx can result in globus pharyngeus, which is the medical term for having a sensation of a lump in the throat (9). The sensation is most notable between swallows. EOR is the most common underlying factor, although other anatomical, physiological, and psychological factors should be considered.

Enlarged Tonsils

Enlarged adenoids, which can block the nasal airway, may also be attributable to EER in very young children. In a study of children less than two years old who underwent surgery for removal of enlarged adenoids, 42% also had a GERD diagnosis.

201

By contrast, GERD was diagnosed in only 7% of a control group of children getting surgery for insertion of ear tubes but whose adenoids were normal. The association between reflux and adenoid enlargement was even stronger in children age one or less. In this age group, 88% of those requiring adenoidectomy had a GERD diagnosis, whereas only 14% of the control group getting ear tubes had a GERD (21) diagnosis.

Rhinosinusitis (Nose & Sinus Infection)

Reflux may be a factor in inflammation of the nose and sinuses. Called rhinosinusitis, this inflammation is caused by obstruction of the final common pathway of the maxillary, ethmoid, and frontal sinus tracts. Although infection is often present, it is not typically the primary underlying factor for rhinosinusitis. Rather, infection occurs secondarily because the impaired drainage due to swelling, or oedema, of sinus and nasal tissues creates an ideal environment for the growth of bacteria.

Anything irritating the sinus and nasal tissues can result in swelling of tissues: allergies, cigarette smoke, recurrent viral infections, and EER. Oedema from EER is a common cause of sinus obstruction (22). Another study by Bothwell et al. (23)

found that 89% of children who underwent reflux therapy in addition to maximal medical management of allergy and other irritants could avoid sinus surgery.

Otitis Media (Middle Ear Infection)

*Like the sinuses, the ear has natural openings that must remain functional to prevent problems. As in rhino sinusitis, the development of middle ear infections (otitis media) is a secondary complication that results from impaired function of the Eustachian tube. Studies using animal models have shown that exposure of the middle ear and the Eustachian tube to acid and pepsin results in failure of the Eustachian tube to perform its dual function of sweeping out secretions and modulating pressure within the ear **(24, 25).** In a study examining patients who had chronic ear problems, treatment with the anti-reflux medication omeprazole resulted in complete resolution of symptoms (26).*

Conclusion

EOR is a topic to be investigated along with other important causes of ENT problems such as allergies, immune deficiency, smoke exposure, and other yet-to-be defined factors. EOR is sometimes a difficult diagnosis to make and is even more difficult if not suspected. However, if EOR is discovered to be an underlying or contributing problem, instituting reflux therapy can often control or even eliminate symptoms altogether. (MARCI-Kids.com, 2007)

The full list of the medical references used within this MARCI Kids excerpt is also provided in a separate Appendix in the back of this book[56]

---

[56] For more information and to access the list of references indexed in the above excerpt please use this link: http://web.archive.org/web/20081120220009/http://www.marci-kids.com/eerreferences.html#19

Chapter 14

Sandifers Syndrome

"Sandifers Syndrome[57] is most commonly mistaken for seizures. The child typically appears to have an alteration in mental status associated with the tonic posturing.

- *A relationship with feeding may suggest a diagnosis of Sandifers Syndrome, which commonly occurs after feeding.*

The child may have a sudden rotation of the head and neck to one side and the legs to the opposite side with a stretched out appearance. Typically, the back is arched posteriorly with hyperextension of the spine and elbows may be flexed and held posteriorly with hyperextended

---

[57] Pegeen Eslami, M. A. P. o. P. D. o. P. E. M. U. M. M. C., 1994-2014 . *Sandifer's Syndrome Clinical Presentation.* [Online] Available at: http://emedicine.medscape.com/article/931761-clinical [Accessed 24 May 2014].

hips. *Torticollis may be present. Although the intermittent stiff tonic posture and periods of crying and apparent discomfort may suggest seizures, in many cases the rhythmic clonic component, which may be present in seizures, is not described.*

- *Various stiff, bizarre postures can be observed.*
- *Typically, the duration of the posture is 1-3 minutes.*
- *This brief, paroxysmal pattern of posturing accounts for the fact that the movement observed in Sandifers Syndrome may be mistaken for seizures.*
- *During the posture, the infant may become very quiet or, less commonly, become very fussy. Fussiness and evident discomfort is most commonly observed as the posture abates*
- *If a significant volume of gastro-oesophageal reflux is observed, even without actual vomitus, some infants and children may manifest evidence of respiratory tract irritation as well, including cough, wheezing, and stridor, depending on the degree and volume of reflux."*
- *My first child born with reflux had Sandifers syndrome. Ryan would fling his arms outstretched, go stiff as a board and turn his head to one side; his eyes would also seem to be in a fixed stare position. This would occur most days and last for a few seconds"*

While Sandifers in a baby is terrifying to watch, it is apparently harmless and causes no harm to the child. This reaction is actually the body's response to protect the baby and momentarily freeze the pain.

Always double check and advise your medical team about any of the changes you may observe in your baby's behaviour, as Sandifers Syndrome can sometimes mimic other health issues.

Chapter 15

Sensory Processing Difficulties & GORD

For a short period of time we felt our nightmare was finally over, however, things started to take a turn for the worst when Raven approached her first birthday. As mentioned previously, before her first birthday, Raven's health started to deteriorate. Over a period of nearly four months she had bronchitis, tonsillitis, acute tonsillitis and ear infections resulting in a burst eardrum.

Raven went off her feeds and started to wake constantly at night and would be wide awake at 4 a.m. every morning. Her crèche started to see a serious decline in her eating and sleeping habits, she would also lash out at other children. Raven could go all day without sleep and food and her behaviour was very challenging. She could not focus on anything and seemed to have a need to be in constant motion.

Raven has now been diagnosed with sensory processing difficulties and has been thoroughly assessed by two different services resulting in this diagnosis.

I feel her early childhood trauma and difficulties with feeding have had a serious impact in the way she presents today. I also feel she always had underlying issues which made GORD even harder for her to deal with and process. A mother's gut feelings are seldom wrong.

Excerpt from on Call Children's Therapy Network[58]

Dr Fiona Jones

"Sensory processing difficulties appear to be common for children with reflux. Approximately 51% of children with reflux also present with a major feeding difficulty such as food refusal, food selectivity, dysphagia or poor oral motor skills. It is interesting to note that 93% of feeding difficulties are found to result from a combination of organic causes (such as reflux) and

---

[58] Jones Dr Fiona , On Call Children's Therapy Network, Suite 6, Leve1 1 Kenmore Village, Kenmore, Queensland, Australia) Phone: 07 3378 9543, Fax: 07 3878 5144 Email: admin@occtherapy.com.au Postal Address: PO Box 1118, Kenmore QLD 4069

secondary behavioural characteristics (such as avoiding meal times).

Many children with reflux also have sensory processing difficulties. Sensory processing is the process of taking in, organising and responding to the information we receive through our senses. There are 8 primary senses through which the body receives information:

1. *Visual (see)*
2. *Auditory (hear)*
3. *Tactile (touch)*
4. *Gustatory (taste)*
5. *Olfactory (smell)*
6. *Vestibular (moving)*
7. *Proprioceptive (body awareness and muscle feedback)*
8. *Internal senses (e.g. hunger, thirst, temperature)*

Everyone processes sensory information differently but some have more difficulty than others dealing with certain types of sensory information and creating an appropriate response. There are four main patterns of behavioural responses to sensory input, as described below.

Level of Input Required to Register High (Under-Sensitive), Low Registration

The degree to which a person misses sensory input: 'What's happening?

Positives:

- *Easy going*
- *"Go with the flow"*

Can be difficult:

- *To get started*
- *To tune in during class*

To change speeds (often work at the same pace even if the family is in a rush)

Sensation Seeking

The degree to which a person obtains sensory input; I like it and I want more', 'on the go'

Positives:

- *Good multi-tasker*
- *Adventurous*

Can be difficult:

- *To stay on task (often procrastinate)*
- *To calmly and quietly sit and listen without fidgeting*

Low Sensitivity to Stimuli

The degree to which a person detects sensory input: 'This bothers me'

Positives:

- *More perceptive*
- *Higher problem solving ability*
- *Notice the finer details*

Can be difficult:

- *Social situations can be more challenging*
- *Seeing the bigger picture*
- *Trying new activities*

Sensation Avoiding

The degree to which a person is bothered by sensory input: 'I must get away from this'

Positives:

- Good at designing and implementing structure and routines
- Can be difficult:

To stay calm and concentrate in new or unpredictable environments

Children may have different responses at different times of the day, and for different senses. For example, one might be hypersensitive to taste and texture, but seek movement (vestibular)."

How Does Sensory Processing work?

All sensory information (sight, taste, smell, touch, sound, hunger, movement, etc.) is initially processed at the brainstem m, which *works like a filter. Important information is sent through to the cortex of the brain for processing, whereas insignificant sensory input (i.e. weak, repetitive or familiar input) is filtered out. This happens at a reflex level – it is not something that you think about. This keeps the cortex, or "thinking part" of the brain, free to process new information or to think about what you are doing. Sometimes, the brainstem does not filter sensory information effectively, and may filter out important information mistakenly.*

Once information has passed through the filter, it will go to either the "processing centre" or the "danger centre". If sensory information is sent to the "danger centre", this helps the body get ready to respond. Your body may then be ready for fight, flight (run), fright (scare) or freeze. This response releases adrenaline into the system to prepare the body and to respond.i

EXAMPLE (Adrenaline Response)

If you put your hand on something burning, this information is sent straight to the "danger centre" in the brain, adrenaline is released, and you will respond instantly (e.g. flight – pulling your hand back). This is a protective response that helps our bodies get out of dangerous situations quickly, without needing to think about what to do.

When your body goes into an adrenaline response, you are unable to accurately think and process information. This means that if your child goes into "fight or flight" then it will be very difficult to reason with him/her until they have calmed down. In fact, they may not be able to process anything that is said to them during this time. It can take children quite a while to calm down, and if they are not fully calm before returning to task, they are far more likely to reach a meltdown stage again quickly.

Sometimes, our bodies remember something that felt uncomfortable a long time ago. It sends this information to the danger centre. This means that children can have this protective adrenaline response to sensory information that other people perceive as being safe and normal (or even unnoticed!). For example, think of how you might react if you hear a squealing tyre after a recent car accident.

Consequently, children with reflux may develop a sensory and emotional aversion to eating. They often experience hypersensitivity to the sensory components of eating, such as taste, texture (e.g. lumps in puree), changes in appearance or temperature of their food, or the feeling of food on their lips or hands. Their experience of eating may be linked with activation of their 'danger centre' due to the pain and discomfort associated with reflux. This may contribute to ongoing gagging, vomiting and food avoidance.

Children may then rely on predictability, routine, distraction and control to eat.

The management goals for children with reflux are typically focused on:

1. *Medical management to reduce vomiting, pain and discomfort.*
2. *Rebuilding trust and confidence in eating by making it a pleasurable and safe experience.*
3. *Develop oral skills.*
4. *Decrease hypersensitive gagging and vomiting reflexes.*
5. *Reduce the emotion and stress level.*

What Can You Do?

Speak with an occupational therapist or speech pathologist for assistance:

1. Start with "safe" feeding experiences, and change or add one small step at a time (e.g. change the appearance of

2. The puree by putting it in a different bowl or eating it with a rusk stick as a spoon).

3. Engage your child in messy play with or without food. For example, you could finger paint with puree or make people out of food items.

4. Recognise the small steps. Smelling a new food (even if they don't eat it) is a step toward feeling secure enough to taste it.

5. Encourage, but never force, the next step toward eating. If your child will allow a new food on their plate, you may like to encourage them to play with it, or give it a kiss.

6. When they are comfortable doing so, you can encourage them to lick the food or taste and spit it out".

Chapter 16

GORD and Emotions - The Personal Side

Living with a baby with severe GORD is extremely hard on relationships and marriages are rocked to the core. Everything you hoped and dreamed of while pregnant is suddenly lost in the midst of pain and suffering. You long for the baby you dreamed of. Happiness can seem like a distant memory. I remember many nights sitting on my own crying and asking, why us?

It seemed so unfair. I would see other mothers enjoying their babies and having normal lives.

At one stage I lost all my body hair from stress. I was drained, days turned into weeks, weeks turned into months and still the nightmare was never-ending. The lack of sleep was the worst; everything seemed to multiply when I was tired. Some days I actually felt like I could not go on, no one seemed to understand.

Eventually friends stopped calling, family stayed away and I was left alone with my screaming baby in so much pain and there was nothing I could do and no one to turn too. Doctors and hospitals had no answers for me; it was like they didn't care.

When Raven was about 4 months old I couldn't handle the screams in the house anymore, the walls seemed to close in on me. I wrapped Raven up and put her into her pram and went out for a walk in the torrential rain, I didn't care I had no rain clothes or umbrella. I let the rain soak me to the bone, my own hot tears streamed down my face. I pounded that path like it was reflux, every stomp; every stride I took seemed to work the anger out of me. I wanted the world to know how I was feeling. I hoped that some stranger might stop me and ask was I ok? Could they help?

I just wanted to connect with someone.

Reflux had us broke at this stage, Lee was in college I couldn't return to work. We where now living of my credit card and lee's back to education allowance. Financial stress, my other two children to think about, a baby that never stopped screaming, pressure from medical professionals, who constantly scrutinised our parenting. I felt I was ready to buckle.

As my mind swirled into oblivion, I pushed the pram through the doors of the local social welfare office to ask had our application for financial

219

assistance been accepted. The woman in reception looked down her nose at me like I was a drenched rat with a screaming infant in the pram. I was visibly upset but she never asked me was I ok, instead she took great delight in telling me that myself and my husband didn't qualify for assistance because we earned too much, at that stage we where surviving on 360 euro a week for a family of 5. That day is etched in my mind as being the final straw. If you have ever heard of marathon runners getting a second wind I got mine that day and set up my group.

GORD is a very scary world to be trapped in. This is why I vowed to do something productive. I wanted to gain something from this negative experience and turn it around. I didn't want all this suffering and heart ache to be for nothing. When I set up my group, one by one these amazing mothers flooded in. All of us suffering the same pain, all of us having this connection that only a mother of a reflux baby understands.

I hope in writing this book I can help others by passing on the experience and advice, the mistakes and successes that I have learned along the way. My mission is to try and spare any parent from months of anguish. Above all I want to reach out to anyone suffering this alone.

The following Beautiful Stories Have Been Shared With Me From the Wonderful, Powerful Mothers of Surviving Reflux Ireland

Mother 1

"My story doesn't compare with some of you mammies, as I feel that we got sorted with the correct meds/feed balance. My advice would be to speak up for your little baby as soon as you can. If you feel that there's something not right, then you're probably right."

Mother 2

"I knew in the hospital that my baba was puking up most feeds, only to be fobbed off time & time again. Because of the lack of continuity with care over the Christmas period, we had a crap Christmas! A far cry from the 'ah isn't it lovely to have your little baby here for Christmas' that we heard over & over!!!

My baba couldn't lie flat & only wanted to be held, which also resulted in the 'oh she's getting spoilt' comments. I think people should be more sensitive to people who've just had babies & not presume that it's as simple as the textbook. I found it very difficult to get info on formula choices too, which is something that I found infuriating! This resulted in numerous tins of wasted powders & disappointing results. I really feel for people who haven't found the help that they need for their baby, no matter what the balance of meds/feeds etc. is. My little one is almost 6 months now & I'm really enjoying her now, but the first 3 months were so hard. Keep up the good work & speak up for your baby, if u don't then nobody else will x".

Mother 3

"After 9 months we finally have a happy baby. It's been a long road, doctors, paeds, osteopathy, chiropractor, faith-healers and numerous "cures", nine different formulas, Losec and Gaviscon. Reflux has ruled our house and affected our little family. It has cut us off from family, friends and social events. It turned me into a wreck so exhausted and sleep deprived that on one rare occasion that I had to leave the house with a screaming baby and cranky toddler in toe, I was so flustered that I reversed into a bollard, so I'm blaming reflux for that costly repair too. It robbed me of my confidence as a mother that I was failing my little girl.

I've cried a tsunami never mind a river over the months. Finally it's all coming good and we're getting our lives back on track and enjoying our little girl who is now off meds apart from Gaviscon in 2 bottles a day and has a good variety of foods she can tolerate. We have the odd bad day when teething causes a flare up. Without this page and the wisdom of the mammies on it I would still be clueless as to how to help my little girl. It has been my bible and you Cherie Bacon as I've said before are the Mother Teresa of Reflux Mammies xx".

Mother 4

"I had a year of hell with silent reflux on my first, I knew something was wrong, but was told it's just colic, brought him to hospital after he had only taken 7 oz. in 24 hrs and was told I probably wasn't feeding him right, I was a nervous first time mother and from someone I thought was a good friend I was told get over it, all babies cry, you're just being dramatic!!!! I went privately to the children's practice with my little list of problems and was nearly afraid to talk because I thought they would say the same, she told me to read the list and after 3 things asked me what I thought it was, and when she said you're right, a mother always knows, I started to cry because finally someone

had listened. It took Nutramigen, Zantac and Losec together to get it under control, had major flares from some foods, there was a time I thought I'd never be able to bring him out in public and I lost 3 friends who were horrible to me during that time but we got through it thankfully and I have a very happy 3 year old now, as well as a 4 month old, busy house here".

Mother 5

"My story is pretty much the same as yours. Having a premature baby with his own challenges and first op soon after he was born was hard dealing with it. He was such a happy little guy, slept woke ate slept woke ate giggled after 6wks. He was diagnosed with silent reflux after a short stay in hospital; it changed our lives for the worse. After 10+formulas, countless meds and dosage changes, still everything is as bad as ever. Cranial didn't help; just put a bigger hole in our pocket.

The baby slept in 45min intervals round the clock, he screamed constantly and still have hours of it per day although he's sleeping 3-4hrs at night when put up after midnight. Its horrible waking constantly at 8mths, it's exhausting. I'm crying constantly, I feel helpless and so alone. My toddler is suffering and getting cheeky because he craves attention which I can't give anymore and my relationship suffers. I can't go places and I can't leave him with anyone for fear they won't be able to settle the baby. It's ruined any happiness I've ever had. I've been living in an endless nightmare, like you say nobody understands how hard it is.

I've been and still get to an all-time low where I have to debate with myself if I should continue and if my boys could be ok without me in this life. I constantly have this battle and the isolation you feel is so depressing".

Mother 6

"I just want to say that there is light at end of tunnel. Had Sam for paed check-up this week and she's recommending we come off the thickened formula - we gave him a bottle of cow's milk Tues night & touch wood no issues! - We were last with her in November and she recommended coming off Losec then, and also no issues.

I think we're finally there (I whisper to you all!), after having bad silent reflux from day 1, leading to very bad respiratory issues, *aspiration, 6 stays in hospital including an ambulance dash from Portlaoise to Dublin & a few nights in Temple St ICU, my chest pumping him on the hall floor, cranial therapists, quacks, consultants - then finally to this little pudding that fills our lives with joy every day!*

Despite all his prodding & poking (he's been tested for everything as he also is long sighted & has hearing issues despite there being neither in our families' history) he is the happiest, smiley baby you'll ever meet - and clearly I'm not biased. There is hope!"

Mother 7

"My reflux story...My husband and I were over the moon when we discovered I was expecting our first baby. We were so excited and a little nervous as we ventured into the unknown having previously had very little exposure to babies!

Our beautiful baby boy was born on August 13th 2013 ten days earlier than expected. My plans were to breastfeed my baby, what is supposed to be the most natural thing in the world. This was extremely painful and didn't seem to be working. Midwives came and went and each one poked and prodded at me to get the baby to latch on. Bit by bit I began to lose confidence in my ability to breastfeed and I was worried sick that my baby wasn't feeding enough as he would latch off after a few minutes.

After 3 days of this I made the decision to switch to formula. On the second day of giving formula (my son was 5 days old at this stage) we had a terrifying incident where he projectile vomited his bottle all over the place. We were advised to change his formula and this was the start of what was to come.

By the time he was 10 days old he had diarrhoea, red hives and a severe nappy rash developing. I wondered if these symptoms were due to a milk allergy as I knew I was CMPI as an infant plus we have a history of allergies on my side of the family. These symptoms were all dismissed and I was told the diarrhoea was because he was on comfort formula, the hives were milk spots and his nappy rash was very common for a baby of his age.

This continued along with several formula changes and by the time he was three and a half weeks old the screaming started – inconsolable and endless screaming. This went on for hours and hours on end. No matter what we did it would not stop and we felt as helpless as we had no idea what was going on.

The screaming then developed at night time and my husband and I would take turns walking the floors trying to stop the crying. It was heart-breaking and we were just about existing ourselves between physical and mental exhaustion coupled with stress, worry and anxiety about our baby being in pain - it was so tough. Nothing was working.

At about 9 weeks old we finally cut a break but then he developed bronchiolitis at 10 weeks old which landed him in hospital for 10 days. The next few months passed in a complete blur of sleepless nights, horrendous days and we became prisoners in our own home. The stares from people if we ventured out on a rare occasion were enough to prevent us putting a foot outside the door the next time.

We had seven and a half horrific months of horrible, disgusting reflux at its worst. During this time, we were met with complete ignorance and lack of awareness amongst the medical profession about this condition and were constantly being dismissed and treated like we were just over-reactive first-time parents. The whole thing took its toll on our relationship and we used to bark at each other instead of speaking. Exhaustion made our brains fuzzy and we had no life outside our home.

Looking back now - my husband was amazing and did so much to try and help me but unfortunately, no matter how much he did - it was never enough. I wanted the pain to go away and to find a cure for our poor helpless little baby.

I spent every waking hour I could on the net researching and looking for answers as to why my baby was experiencing this excruciating pain that despite being on adequate medication - it still was far from under control. By this stage we had made 5 attempts to wean him and each one ended with him having severe non IgE mediated reactions, which in turn, drove his reflux crazy for days on end.

The horrible thing was - despite having photographic and video evidence, nobody in the medical profession believed us about the severity of what was happening. Instead we were made fun of and felt like we were making it all up. We were poked fun at which left us feeling like we had been punched in the stomach. All we wanted was help and support to find out what was wrong.

We eventually got a referral to another hospital and around the same time I came across a drug that was being used on babies in the UK having similar reactions to food that our little man was having. I did my research and was armed with information for my first encounter with our allergist paediatrician.

At last we met someone that cared and listened and despite having never heard of using Ketotifen for gut inflammation, she agreed to trial him on it. We had the most amazing 4 weeks of normality after introducing Ketotifen. Our baby increased his intake tenfold of his formula and the squealing stopped. He started sleeping through the night and we began to lead a normal life and do normal things like go for coffee in a coffee shop without people staring disapprovingly at our screaming baby. At eight and a half months old, we introduced weaning again and it was here that we discovered our baby had a rare condition called FPIES (Food Protein Induced Enterocolitis syndrome) when he experienced an acute reaction to avocado. We are now at ten months and currently have two safe foods - soya formula and oats.

To say it has been an emotional rollercoaster would be an absolute understatement. Our lives have been turned upside down and inside out living with a baby with reflux. It has been the toughest thing I have personally ever had to deal with.

Having a baby with GORD is just completely, totally and utterly soul destroying. We have had to fight and battle every inch of the way to get help and it has been physically, mentally and emotionally exhausting. We have such a long road ahead of us still to go but I will continue to fight every inch of the way to ensure that my son gets cared for until we reach the other side.

I thank God every day that my son does not have a life-threatening illness and he will one day be a healthy little boy.

But it doesn't make the journey we have to undertake in order to get there, any easier. I am also very thankful for the Surviving Reflux Ireland page which I have gained so much help and support from. It helps to know we are not alone and there are other people out there experiencing similar setbacks. I honestly do not know how we would have got through the dark days without it.

This whole experience has completely affected me personally. It has rocked me to my inner core and all my self-belief has gone from not being heard when I was screaming for help. My main priority at the minute is my gorgeous little baby and 'fixing' him and then I hope to get my own life back on track.

I just want to say to any mother out there living with GORD - do not give up. Keep fighting for your baby as you are their voice and your gut instinct will never ever let you down. It's ALWAYS right. Talk to your partner and try to keep communication lines open at all times as you need each other to get through this.

Don't be afraid to ask for help from family members - it is impossible to do it alone and always trust the advice given on the page as the ladies on it know more than any medical professional I've ever met!!!!!! Xxx".

Fathers' Voices

Most often a father's struggle is rarely recognized within a family who is confronted with a child with reflux. Often these men are the backbone of the family and take the brunt of the situation.

Mothers seem to have the luxury of being able to vocalize their fear, frustrations and concerns to each other and within the support groups on social media platforms.

Sadly, matters have not changed much over the years for men, their voices are not recognized and they are marginalized within society, when it comes to parental matters. Speaking about one's feelings is not an option and is not acceptable. Often these men suffer in silence and are never heard.

Here are a few sentiments and experiences shared with me by fathers of children with reflux.

Father 1

'Having a child with reflux is the hardest and most painful thing a man/father can physically go through. I often thought to myself when will this end when will the crying and hurting stop. Men are typically strong when it comes to the emotional side of life, but I can say that emotions got the better of me on this one. I along with my wife, were emotional wrecks by the 5th month of my daughter's existence in the world.

My daughter was my 1st child and when she was born, I was overjoyed with happiness at the sight of her. After 2 days myself and my wife both said to each other that she was the best baby, we had ever heard of, as all she did was eat and sleep. I thought to myself what a model baby, how we were so lucky to get such a good child, as you would always hear the stories of babies crying nonstop. I thought to myself, I wouldn't like to be in that position. The best baby, we had ever heard off! Well, that was all about to change.

The emotional roller coaster of a life with a reflux baby reared its ugly head by day 3 of my daughter's life. This was the beginning of what I can only describe as the toughest 2 years of my lifetime.

The crying and screaming from the acid burn that my daughter experienced, started out as a minor issue, which we believed was a spell of colic.

We soon realized, after many hospital visits that this was not the case. I used to leave in the morning with my daughter crying with the pain, only to return home later that night to the exact situation. The pain never seemed to ease or stop and this carried on for 5 months continuously without a break.

As a man you are brought up thinking that your task is to be the primary provider for your family, protect the women and kids.

How could I protect my daughter from such a serious illness, even the hospitals and doctors knew so little about the true nature of this disease and the impact it has on a family. How could I protect my wife from the worries and struggles she dealt with on a daily basis while I went off to college.

Now don't get me wrong, I had done my fair share of duties as a father, but I must commend my wife during this time, she was seriously strong willed and kept things going.

Life was a serious battle for the first two years of my daughter's life. When she was at her worst we had to move her downstairs to the back room and would take turns minding her in shifts.

I used to pity my wife so much when she was on the night shift, as I used to get sleep and head off to college, knowing full well that she was stuck there all day, absolutely exhausted after having no sleep all night.

No matter what we tried nothing ever seemed to work. I used to think we were going crazy and why this was happening to us, had we not suffered enough.

Every time we would visit the doctors or hospital we would get the same old lines, about how we should just wait and see, that things will improve when the baby is 2 months, it's just colic, it will pass, wait till she reaches 4 months and starts on the solids that things will get much better, wait till she's walking, the list went on and on.

I remembered how she used to present beautifully at all the doctor's visits. This made me get extremely annoyed, as we wanted to get to the bottom of what was going on and we knew we needed to get some answers to save our sanity.

I thought the older she got the better she would be, but the food seemed to make her worse in all aspects. I didn't know how much more of this I could take.

The endless battle with baby formulas and foods continued for two years of my daughter's life, she had allergies and had reactions to most foods. They seemed to flare the reflux. It was so hard to judge what foods were causing the reflux and which foods were safe.

Slowly but surely myself and my wife started to drift apart, as I'm sure most couples who have a reflux baby do, as there is no real closeness any more. Both of us were totally exhausted and basically had no time for each other as all our waking day and nights focused on our daughters well being.

Many people say when your baby sleeps you sleep, but with a reflux baby this is not the case because reflux babies do not sleep. How could they with a raging inferno burning away in their chest. No sleep leads to exhaustion which leads to constant fighting. All this can result in jealously as when one is fresher than the other; ultimately it can make the strongest of marriages to crumble.

Father 2

"Unless your living under the same roof as a reflux baby, people just don't understand. It really makes me laughs when people who have no children tell me how tired they are. I do think that because our 2 were\are such bad sleepers they were developmentally months ahead of themselves. 3yr old had unreal speech very early on. She walked at 10.5mths and potty trained herself just before 2yrs. The almost 10mth old is already pulling herself up with a few weeks. Being up at 5am every morning with her means I spend more time with her I suppose even though it is very draining sometimes. It causes a lot of stress in our house and I don't want to wish the time away but I look forward to the day where I don't see 5am".

Father 3

Dad to a 2 year old little boy (hard core refluxer) and 6 month old girl (mild reflux)

"It's not easy being a dad. Witnessing childbirth for the first time is traumatic enough and having a new baby home is a major change but nothing had prepared me for reflux.

It was horrible. When I'd come home from work I would find my worn out wife and new baby boy both crying, having been like that pretty much all day. It broke me seeing him in pain like that. We did everything we could to give him an ease from it. We slept in a separate room, took it in turns so that one of us slept while the other would let him sleep upright in our arms.

I've no idea how I managed to pull myself together for work every day. As a reflux dad you have to deal with dismissive doctors, your partner turning into a wreck, your baby being in near constant pain, you still have to face into work every day and unfortunately the only consolation I have to offer other reflux dads is that it ends eventually."

Father 4

"Shane used to always say to Harry over and over again when he was screaming in his arms at night!"I won't give up on you"".

Father 5

"My husband said his main feelings about our little girl having reflux and cmpi was frustration. He's not Irish and he couldn't get

over how dismissive a doctor could be of parents concerns about their baby.

Being fobbed off all the time he was really frustrated with the doctors. He felt it wasn't just my responsibility to sort it out and felt he had to take time off work and come with me to our Gp and fight with me to have her put onto Zantac and then losec and fight for them to listen to us.

At times he said he felt helpless and wondered how we were going to get through it, but we'd been through hard times before and this wasn't going to break us! He felt like if we could laugh at least once a day he had done his job hence the song about smelly Nutramigen".

A Parent Doing the Job Alone

"When I first heard of reflux in babies, I was told that symptoms are vomiting/spiting up, poor feeding habits, crankiness and poor sleeping. I was prepared for sleepless nights anyway, but I wasn't prepared for the damage that it does to you emotionally. Now that may sound dramatic to someone who hasn't raised a reflux baby, but if you have you know what I mean by this.

The screaming of pain when you try do a normal thing like give them a bottle, the arching of the back when their pulling away from you and all your trying to do is nourish their tiny body is truly heartbreaking. You feel nobody understands, and the truth is there are few around you that do. Your doctors or health nurses pawn you off as a paranoid mother and assure you your baby is "thriving". You will come to hate the word thriving believe me.

I am ashamed to admit that I hated life for months. I thought the painful cries of my baby and the looks from passersby staring at you with judgemental faces wondering why you can't console your baby would never end. I didn't go outside the door for days I could not bear it. On top of this you are physically exhausted from doing everything bar standing on your head to try keeping your baby happy. But one day while I was back at my GP (for the 20th time) I just couldn't hold in my emotions and the floodgates opened.

I cried my heart and soul out to the woman and she placed her hand on my shoulder and said its time now to sort all this out. And that's when my baby was finally put on medication, after weeks of trying things like comfort formula, gripe water, cot propping, I was finally prescribed medications my child desperately needed. It was like a huge weight lifted and I finally felt someone listened to me.

The week she started the meds was still tough but after about 4 days my child was like a new girl. She still was wary of bottles but the change in her personality was incredible and she smiled her adorable chubby cheeked smile more and more as the days went on. We went out more and I felt more confident in myself as a woman and as a mother.

I did all of this on my own with the help of no man. So to anyone out there who is raising a reflux baby alone, don't worry. You will get there someday and I promise you things get better. It may take a month or even a year, but never lose the faith and know each time you pick up the phone to hassle your doctor you are doing this out of love for your child. There is light at the end of the tunnel. I promise."

Chapter 17

Useful Financial Assistance for Parents Living in Ireland

All information provided is accurate at the time of print

There may be circumstances where parents can apply for financial medical assistance.

This section of the book contains some collaborated information which has been provided by the *Citizens Information* website in Ireland; other countries may have the same assistance so please check your local advice center.

Maternity Leave

If you become pregnant while in employment, you are entitled to take maternity leave. The entitlement to a basic period of maternity leave from employment extends to all female employees (including casual workers), regardless of how long you have been working for the organisation or the number of hours worked per week. You can also avail of additional unpaid maternity leave.

The *Maternity Protection Acts 1994 and 2004* provide your statutory minimum entitlements in relation to maternity at work including maternity leave.

You are entitled to 26 weeks' maternity leave together with 16 weeks additional unpaid maternity leave, which begins immediately after the end of maternity leave.

Under the *Maternity Protection (Amendment) Act 2004* at least 2 weeks have to be taken before the end of the week of your baby's expected birth and at least 4 weeks after. You can decide how you would like to take the remaining weeks. Generally, employees take 2 weeks before the birth and the remaining weeks after. If you qualify for Maternity Benefit (see below) at least 2 and no more than 16 weeks must be taken before the end of the week the baby is due.

Father's Entitlement to Maternity Leave

Fathers are entitled to maternity leave if the mother dies within 40 weeks of the birth. In these circumstances, the father is entitled to a period of leave, the extent of which depends on the actual date of the mother's death. If the mother dies within 24 weeks of the birth, he has an optional right to the additional maternity leave. If the mother's death is over 24 weeks after the birth, the father is entitled to leave until 40 weeks after the birth. The leave starts within 7 days of the mother's death.

Paternity Leave

Paternity leave is not recognised in employment law. In other words, employers are not obliged to grant male employees special paternity leaves (either paid or unpaid) following the birth of their child. Annual leave taken following the birth of a child is treated in employment law in the same way as leave taken at any other time of the year. It is at the discretion of the employer to decide who can and cannot take annual leave at a given time.

Some employers, (for example, the civil service), do provide a period of paid leave from work for male employees following the birth or adoption of their child. Fathers employed in the civil service are entitled to a period of special (paternal) leave of 3 days with pay in respect of children born on or after 1 January, 2000 or for children adopted after 1 January 2000.

The employee usually applies for this leave in writing before the birth or adoption. Arrangements where employers provide this type of leave following the birth or adoption of a child are the result of negotiation and agreement reached between the employer and employee. These arrangements are not covered by employment law so if an employer agrees to provide time off to an employee as paternal leave for a specified period (either with or without pay), it is entirely discretionary.

While male employees are not entitled under law to either paid or unpaid paternity leave, they may be entitled to parental leave. Parental leave entitles both parents who qualify to take a period of up to 18 weeks' unpaid leave from employment in respect of children up to 8 years of age.

A two week provision for paid paternity leave is currently being drafted and will be included in the family Leave Bill.

The Bill will consolidate current provisions for maternity, adoptive, parental and carers' leave into one piece of legislation.

Postponing Maternity Leave

Section 7 of the Maternity Protection (Amendment) Act 2004 provides for postponement of maternity leave in strict circumstances, that is, if your baby is hospitalised. This right to postpone leave applies whether you are on maternity leave, or on additional unpaid maternity leave. Note, your employer has the right to refuse your application to postpone your maternity leave. There are details about postponing maternity leave in 'Further information' can be found on the link below[59].

Parental Leave

The *Parental Leave Act 1998* as amended by the *Parental Leave (Amendment) Act 1998*, allows parents to take parental leave from employment in respect of certain children. A person acting in loco parentis with respect to an eligible child is also eligible.

---

[59]http://www.citizensinformation.ie/en/employment/employment_rights_and_conditions/leave_and_holidays/maternity_leave.html

Extension of Parental Leave to 18 weeks

On 8 March 2013 the *European Union (Parental Leave) Regulations 2013* increased the amount of parental leave available to each parent per child from 14 weeks to 18 weeks. (Those who have taken or are taking 14 weeks' parental leave are also entitled to this extra 4 weeks.) The Regulations extended the age limit for a child with a long-term illness to 16 years. They also provide that a parent returning from parental leave may request a change in working hours – see 'Rules' below. The Regulations apply to all children who qualify for parental leave.

Age of Child

Since 18 May 2006, leave can be taken in respect of a child up to 8 years of age. If a child was adopted between the age of 6 and 8, leave in respect of that child may be taken up to 2 years after the date of the adoption order. In the case of a child with a disability or a long-term illness leave may be taken up to 16 years of age. In addition an extension may also be allowed where illness or other incapacity prevented the employee taking the leave within the normal period.

Amount of Parental Leave

Since 8 March 2013 the amount of parental leave available for each child amounts to a total of 18 working weeks per child. Where an employee has more than one child, parental leave is limited to 18 weeks in a 12-month period. This can be longer if the employer agrees. Parents of twins or triplets can take more than 18 weeks of parental leave in a year.

The 18 weeks per child may be taken in one continuous period or in 2 separate blocks of a minimum of 6 weeks. There must be a gap of at least 10 weeks between the 2 periods of parental leave per child. However, if your employer agrees you can separate your leave into periods of days or even hours.

Both parents have an equal separate entitlement to parental leave. Unless you and your partner work for the same employer, you can only claim your own parental leave entitlement (18 weeks per child). If you both work for the same employer and your employer agrees you may transfer 14 weeks of your parental leave entitlement to each other.

Illness of Parent

If the parent becomes ill while on parental leave and is unable to care for the child the leave can be suspended for the duration of the illness. In order to suspend the parental leave the employee must give written notice and relevant evidence of the illness to the employer as soon as is reasonably practicable. The parental leave resumes after the illness. During the illness the parent is treated as an employee who is sick.

Employment Rights While on Parental Leave

You are not entitled to pay from your employer while you are on parental leave nor are you entitled to any social welfare payment equivalent to *Maternity Benefit or Adoptive Benefit*.

Taking parental leave does not affect other employment rights you have. Apart from the loss of pay and pension contributions, your position remains as if no parental leave had been taken. This means, for example that time spent on parental leave can be used to accumulate your annual leave entitlement.

The legislation only provides for the minimum entitlement. Your contract may give you more extensive rights.

Social Insurance Contributions

The Minister for Social Protection has introduced Regulations to ensure preservation of social insurance (PRSI) records for employees who take parental leave. Your employer must write to the Records Update Section of Department of Social Protection (DSP), detailing the weeks you have not worked, so that you can get *Credited PRSI Contributions* for this time (see 'Where to apply' below). You can find information about *Credited Contributions and Parental Leave* on the DSP website.

Annual Leave and Public Holidays

While on parental leave, you must be regarded for employment rights purposes as still working. This means that you can build up annual leave while on parental leave. If your annual holidays fall due during parental leave, they may be taken at a later time. A public holiday that falls while you are on parental leave and on a day when you would normally be working is added to your period of leave.

Rules

➢ *Generally you must have been working for your employer for a year before you are entitled to parental leave. However if your child is very near the age threshold and you have been working for your employer for more than three months but less than one year you are entitled to pro-rata parental leave. This is one week's leave for every month of employment completed.*

➢ *If you change job and have used part of your parental leave allowance you can use the remainder after one year's employment with your new employer provided your child is still under the qualifying age.*

➢ *Apart from a refusal on the grounds on non-entitlement, an employer may also postpone the leave for up to 6 months. This must be done before the confirmation document is signed. After that, the leave cannot be postponed without further written agreement. Grounds for such a postponement include lack of cover or the fact that other employees are already on parental leave. Normally only one postponement is allowed, but it may be postponed twice if the reason is seasonal variations in the volume of work.*

➤ *Parental leave is to be used only to take care of the child concerned. If the parental leave is taken and used for another purpose the employer is entitled to cancel the leave.*

➤ *Employers must keep records of all parental leave taken by their employees. These records must include the period of employment of each employee and the dates and times of the leave taken. Employers must keep these records for 8 years. If an employer fails to keep records they may be liable to a fine of up to €2000.*

➤ *You are entitled to return to your job after your parental leave unless it is not reasonably practicable for the employer to allow you to return to your old job. If this is the case you must be offered a suitable alternative on terms no less favourable compared with the previous job including any improvement in pay or other conditions which occurred while you were on parental leave.*

➤ *The legislation protects parents who take parental leave from unfair dismissal.*

➤ **Since 8 March 2013,** *when you return to work after taking parental leave, you are entitled to ask for a change in your work pattern or working hours for a set period. Your employer must consider your request but is not obliged to grant it[60].*

---

[60] http://www.citizensinformation.ie/en/employment/employment_rights_and_conditions/leave_and_holidays/parental_leave.html

Medical Cards

If you have a medical card issued by the Health Service Executive HSE you can receive certain health services free of charge. Normally, your dependent spouse or partner and your children are also covered for the same range of health services.

To qualify for a medical card, your weekly income must be below a certain figure for your family size. Cash income, savings, investments and property (except for your own home) are taken into account in the means test[61].

GP Visit Cards

If you do not qualify for a medical card you may be eligible for a GP Visit Card. A GP Visit Card allows you to visit your family doctor for free.

---

[61] http://www.citizensinformation.ie/en/employment/employment_rights_and_conditions/leave_a nd_holidays/parental_leave.html

Unless you have a medical card or a GP Visit Card, visits to family doctors are not free. In order to qualify for a GP Visit Card, you must be ordinarily resident in Ireland. That is, you must be currently living here and intend to continue to live here for a year. You can read more about entitlement to public health services here. You must also meet specific income guidelines.

In situations where, for example, someone has an ongoing medical condition that requires exceptional and regular medical treatment or visits to the doctor, the Health Service Executive (HSE) may grant a Card to that individual or family even where their income is greater than the guidelines. Usually the HSE will only consider these applications where an ongoing medical condition is causing or is likely to cause undue financial hardship.

Having a GP Visit Card only allows you to visit your GP for free. Blood tests to diagnose or monitor a condition are covered but any prescribed drugs associated with your GP visit are not free. Instead, you can apply to become part of the drug payment scheme. The GP Visit Card does not cover hospital charges. It does cover visits to GP out of hour's service.

The GP Visit Card is a plastic card, about the same size as a credit card. It carries your name, your sex, the name of your GP and the validity period of the Card. Cards are subject to review because income levels may change, dependents grow up, or other changes could occur that may affect eligibility.

Budget 2015 included provision for free GP care for all children under 6 years of age and adults aged over 70, to be introduced following negotiations with the Irish Medical Organisation.

Drugs Payment Scheme

Introduction

Under the Drugs Payment Scheme you pay a maximum of €144 a month for approved prescribed drugs; medicines and certain appliances for use by yourself and your family in that month. If a reference price has been set for the drugs you are prescribed, this is the price that the HSE will use to calculate your monthly drugs costs.

Rules

In order to qualify for this scheme, you must be ordinarily resident in Ireland. An ordinarily resident in Ireland means that you have been living here for a minimum of one year or that you intend to live here for a minimum of one year.

The scheme covers the person who applied, his or her spouse/partner, and children aged under 18 (or under 23 if in full-time education). A dependant who is living in the household and has a physical or mental disability or illness and is unable to fully maintain himself/herself, may be included in the family expenditure regardless of age.

When you register for the scheme, your Local Health Office will issue a plastic swipe card for each person named on the registration form. You should present this card whenever you are having prescriptions filled.

Using the Card

You do not have to register with a particular pharmacy for the scheme but for convenience it is advisable to use the same pharmacy in a particular month if you wish to avoid paying more than the maximum €144.

Claiming a Refund for Amounts over the Threshold

If you pay over the maximum, for example, because you need to use two or more pharmacies in one month, you can apply for a refund of the amount above the threshold.

To Apply for a Refund

Get a claim form from your Local Health Office, online at www.drugspayment.ie; or by calling 1890 252 919.

Return the completed claim form to the address given on the form. You can check the status of your application for a refund at www.drugspayment.ie.

Expired Drugs Payment Scheme Cards

Drugs Payment Scheme Cards are issued for a limited time (generally 5 years). When your card expires, you must apply again to obtain a new card. You can get the forms from your local pharmacy or from your Local Health Office.

Lost or Stolen Drugs Payment Scheme Cards

If your Drugs Payment Scheme Card is lost, stolen or damaged, you should contact your Local Health Office[62].

Long Term Illness Scheme

People suffering from certain conditions can get free drugs, medicines and medical and surgical appliances for the treatment of that condition. These are provided under the Long Term Illness Scheme. This scheme is administered by the Health Service Executive (HSE), under *Section 59 Of the Health Act 1970.*

The Long Term Illness Scheme does not depend on your income or other circumstances. You may also be eligible for a Medical Card or GP Visit Card, depending on your circumstances[63].

---

[62] http://www.citizensinformation.ie/en/employment/employment_rights_and_conditions/leave_and_holidays/parental_leave.html
[63] http://www.citizensinformation.ie/en/employment/employment_rights_and_conditions/leave_and_holidays/parental_leave.html

The GMS (Hardship) Assistance

The GMS (Hardship) assistance fund was implemented to cover medical card holders for medication that is not licensed here in Ireland. The non licensed medications such as liquid losec and melatonin will be charged at full price.

When your pharmacist informs you that such medications are not compensated, it is your right to access these through the Hardship Scheme. Your pharmacist will then make an application on your behalf and seek approval from the HSE. Once this has been approved, you do not need to reapply every time you have your prescription filled.

Domiciliary Care Allowance

Domiciliary Care Allowance (DCA) is a monthly payment for a child aged under 16 with a severe disability, who requires ongoing care and attention, substantially over and above the care and attention usually required by a child of the same age. It is not means tested.

You can find the definitions for terms such as severe or substantially in the DCA Medical Guidelines (PDF). These are used by the Department of Social Protection when it is assessing applications for DCA. The guidelines state that the payment is not based on the type of disability, but on the resulting physical or mental impairment which means that the child requires substantially more care and attention than another child of the same age.

The DCA scheme was administered by the Health Service Executive before it was transferred to the Department of Social Protection in 2009.

You can also read the information leaflet form DCA (SW127). The leaflet is available from your Intreo centre or Citizens Information Service[64].

Carer's Allowance

Carer's Allowance is a payment to people on low incomes who are looking after a person who needs support because of age, disability or illness (including mental illness).

If you qualify for a Carer's Allowance you may also qualify for free household benefits (if you are living with the person you are caring for) and a Free Travel Pass. Carer's Allowance is not taken into account in the assessment for a medical card.

---

[64] http://www.citizensinformation.ie/en/employment/employment_rights_and_conditions/leave_and_holidays/parental_leave.html

If you consider that you have been wrongly refused Carer's Allowance, or you are unhappy about a decision of a social welfare deciding officer about your entitlements, you can appeal this decision.

Epilogue

GORD has truly changed my world and how I perceive things.

I will never again judge a mother or any parent. What you see is not always what you get. So many people, who mean well, can say the most hurtful things. When you are so stressed and exhausted and confidence is at an all-time low you can feel like the world is against you.

Thank You for Reading My Book.

Please spread the word with the information you have received.
Together we can change people's perspective of what reflux really is.

We need to change the attitude of:

"It's Only Reflux".

Useful Websites

- ➢ **Infant Acid Reflux App: App for mobile devices**
  https://play.google.com/store/apps/details?id=com.appypie.app ypiea69ea0ddfceb

  https://itunes.apple.com/ie/app/id971312791

- ➢ **The Reflux Bible website**

  http://www.therefluxbible.com

- ➢ **The Reflux Bible Facebook Page: Support page for parents**

  https://www.facebook.com/therefluxbible?ref=hl

- ➢ **Surviving Reflux Ireland: Support group for parents**

  https://www.facebook.com/groups/ RefluxIreland/?fref=ts

- ➢ **Infantreflux.org**

  http://www.infantreflux.org

- ➢ **Reflux Infant Support Association Inc. (RISA)**

  http://www.reflux.org.au/

- ➢ **Infant Acid reflux Solutions: Supplier of TummyCare Max -& BellyBuffers**

  http://www.infant-acid-reflux-solutions.com/

- ➢ **DCA Warrior: Support group for parents**

  https://www.facebook.com/groups/dcawarriors/?fref=ts

263

"The DCA Warriors Group [DCAW] was established in February 2012 to support parents of children with special needs and/or serious illnesses. The co-founders of the group are Ruth Gilhool, Estelle Lewis, Margaret Lennon and Aisling Byrne. Currently DCAW has a membership of approximately 5000 parents. Initially DCAW was mainly focused on providing the members with information and support when applying for Domiciliary Care Allowance, Disability Allowance, Carer's Benefit and Carer's Allowance.

DCAW members are very supportive of each other and the group is known for its confidentiality and the transparency on all areas. As a result of this, the members share and discuss their concerns regarding many areas of their children's lives and needs. In this context, there has been a substantial increase in discussions, seeking of information, offers of support and identification of concerns in relation to members' children with special needs and their education.

DCAW administrators are concerned not only by the volume of the questions raised by members, but also their content. DCAW has carried out surveys and a variety of polls among its members to obtain more information and get a feedback on the provision of support for children with special needs in Ireland's education system. Education has become one of the most important issues and areas of concern for DCAW administrators and members".

➢ *Ruth Gilhool, Co Founder, DCA*

➢ *Lana Mayes: Friend & Reflux book Indi Author*

   http://lanamayes.com/

➢ *Kids with food allergies*

   http://www.kidswithfoodallergies.org/marketplace.html

➢ *MARCI Kids Archived PDF*

   *http://web.archive.org/web/20081120220009/http://www.marc
   i kids.com/eerreferences.html*

➢ *GIKids*

   www.gikids.org

➢ *Reflux Rebels*

   http://www.refluxrebels.com

Indexed References

1. Miedzybrodzka, Z (January 2003). Congenital talipes equinovarus (clubfoot): a disorder of the foot but not the hand. .Journal of anatomy 202 (1): 37–42. PMID 12587918.

2. Patient Education Institute, Treating club foot with Ponseti Treatment,

   www.nlm.nih.gov/medlineplus/tutorials/treatingclubfoot/op

   [Accessed Jan 2015]

3. Lovinsky-Desir, Stephanie MD, Laryngomalacia Medscape Reference, 28 Mar 2014 Available at emedicine.medscape.com/article/1002527-overview. [Accessed June 2014]

4. National Institute for Health and Care Excellence, Gastro-oesophageal reflux disease: recognition, diagnosis and management in children and young people, _2014 Available at http://nice.org.uk/.../gord-in-children-guideline-consultation-draft-nice-gord-in-children-guideline-consultation-draft-nice-guideline2 [Accessed July 2014]

5. American Pregnancy Association, 2014. Colic. [Online] Available at: http://americanpregnancy.org/first-year-of-life/colic/ [Accessed 15 May 2014].

6. Wessel MA, et al. Rule of three: Paroxismal fussing in infancy, sometimes called "colic." Pediatrics. 1954; 14:421-435. Quoted in Birth & beyond/ Colic, American Pregnancy Association Available at http://americanpregnancy.org/first-year-of-life/colic/

7. Colic Calm, 2013-2014. The Cause and Treatment of New-born, Infant and Baby Colic,[Online] Available at: http://www.coliccalm.co.uk/colic.htm [Accessed 6 June 2014]

8. Mersch, John, MD, FAAP. Barium Swallow, Gastroesophageal Reflux (GER and GERD) in Infants and Children, P2. Available at http://www.medicinenet.com/gerd_in_infants_and_children/article.htm [Accessed Feb 2015]

9. Reflux Infants Support Association (RISA) Inc: http://www.reflux.org.au/ [May 15 2014]

10. Mersch, John, MD, FAAP. *Barium Swallow*, Gastroesophageal Reflux (GER and GERD) in Infants and Children, P2. Available at http://www.medicinenet.com/gerd_in_infants_and_children/article.htm [Accessed Feb 2015]

11. Hospital, G.O.S., 2014. Fundoplication - Procedures and treatments, Great Ormond Street Hospital. [Online] Available at: http://www.gosh.nhs.uk/medical-information/procedures-and-treatments/fundoplication/ [Accessed 10 May 2014].

12. Boston Children's Hospital, Esophageal Atresia in Children. Reviewed by Russell W. Jennings, MD© Children's Hospital Boston; posted in 201. Available online at: http://www.childrenshospital.org/conditions-and-treatments/conditions/esophageal-atresia. [Accessed Feb 2015]

13. Suzanne Evans Morris, Ph.D, Children with Feeding Tubes, [online] [Accessed Mar 2015] available at http://www.new-vis.com/fym/papers/p-feed12.htm

14. Web Development © 2007 Invisible Ink, 2007. *Tounge-Tie: From Confusion To Clarity.* [Online] Available at: http://www.tonguetie.net/index.php?option=com_frontpage&Itemid=1 [Accessed 18 May 2014].

15. Weidman Sterling, Evelina, Best-Boss, Angie, Your Child's Teeth: A Complete Guide for Parents . [Online] Available at https://books.google.ie/books?isbn=142141063X - 2013 - Health & Fitness. [Accessed Feb 2015]

16. Udo Erasmus, Fats That Heal, Fats That Kill, Published December 1st 1998 by Alive Books (first published January 1st 1993) Product referred to is UDO'S CHOICE Infant's Blend, GUT MICROFLORA PREPARATION, Information Available at http://.udoschoice.co.uk/products

17. Agency, F. S., Goats' milk formula, not a solution for cows' milk allergic infants. 2014. [Online] Available at: http://www.food.gov.uk/news-updates/news/2014/6003/goats-milk#.U2DtuvIdUko [Accessed 12 May 2014].

18. European Food Safety Authority, Scientific Opinion on the suitability of goat milk protein as a source of protein in infant formulae and in follow-on formulae, EFSA Journal 2012;10(3):2603[18 pp.]. doi:10.2903/j.efsa.2012.2603. Available at http://www.efsa.europa.eu/en/efsajournal/pub/2603.htm

19. GIKids, Digestive Topics: Cow's Milk Protein Intolerance, [Online] Available at: http://www.gikids.org/content/103/en/ [Accessed Feb2015]

20. Vallaeys, Charlotte, DHA and ARA in Infant Formula Dangerous and Unnecessary—Synthetic Additives Have No Place in Infant Foods May 2010—

21. Will Fantle, T. C. I., 2008. DHA/ARA docosahexaenoic acid and arachidonic acid, The Cornucopia Institute, P.O. Box 126, Cornucopia, WI 54827: Will Fantle, The Cornucopia Institute

22. Encyclopaedia Britannica, Faith healing, Definition [Online] Available   at http://www.britannica.com/EBchecked/topic/200569/faith-healing [Accessed Feb 2015]

23. Farlex Partner Medical Dictionary Applied Kinesiology, © Farlex 2012   [Online]   Available   at: http://medicaldictionary.thefreedictionary.com/applied+kinesiol ogy [Accessed 20 April 2014].

24. Farlex Partner Medical Dictionary, therapeutic modality. (N.d. Jonas: Mosby's Dictionary of Complementary and Alternative Medicine. (2005). Available at: http://medical-dictionary.thefreedictionary.com/therapeutic+modality [Accessed April 2014]

25. Nambudripad, Devi S. (2003). NAET: Say Goodbye to Asthma: A Revolutionary Treatment for Allergy-Based Asthma and Other Respiratory Disorders. Say Good-Bye To... Series. Delta Publishing Company. p.37Wikipedia 2014 Nambudripad's Allergy Elimination   Techniques (NAET), http://en.wikipedia.org/wiki/Nambudripad's_Allergy_Eliminatio n_Techniques

26. Bowman, H Naet-Europe [Online] Available at http://www.naet-europe.com/en [Accessed May 17th 2014]

27. MedicineNet, Inc., 1996-2014. Definition of Acupuncture Available at http://www.medicinenet.com/script/main/art.asp?articlekey=2132 [Accessed Feb 2015]

28. Weidman Sterling, Evelina, Best-Boss, Angie, Your Childs Teeth a Complete Guide For Parents Available at https://books.google.ie/books?isbn=142141063X - 2013 - Health & Fitness [Accessed Feb 2015]

29. Murray, Rhona, MPSI, BSc. Pharm Hons Biochemistry M.An.Sc, Health A-Z, Homepharm. Available at: http://www.homepharm.ie/index.php?route=information/nhs/nhs2&id=Osteopathy [Accessed Feb 2015]

30. Irish Association of Craniosacral Therapists, What is Craniosacral Therapy, [online] Available at: http://iacst.ie/craniosacral-therapy. [Accessed Feb 2015]

31. Chiropractic First Dublin, Jan 2015, Chiropractic Adjustment. [Online] Available at: http://www.chiropracticfirstdublin.ie/index.php/chiropractic/ [Accessed Feb 2015]

32. Ketomi Distribution, Colic Calm @2013-2014. Colic Calm. [Online]
Available at: http://www.coliccalm.com.au/blog/cat/baby-colic-gas-reflux [Accessed 12 April 2014].

33. Mc Goldrick, Dorothy, Commonly treated conditions, Colic in Babies, Dunboyne Herbs. Information available at http://www.dunboyneherbs.ie

34. The National Magazine Company Ltd, 2014. NetDoctor.co.uk - The UK's leading independent health website. [Online] Available at: http://www.netdoctor.co.uk/ [Accessed 04 May 2014]

35. Koehn, M., 2011. Help for Acid Reflux, Heartburn, GERD, Indigestion, IBS, Gastro paresis, and Many Other Digestive Issues. [Online] Available at: http://help4acidreflux.wordpress.com/ [Accessed 28 June 2014]

36. Chronic Illness Recovery Counsel Liaison Education, Herxheimer Reaction, [Online] Available at: https://chronicillnessrecovery.org/index.php?option=com_content&view=article&id=161 [Accessed Feb 2015]

37. MedicineNet, Inc., 1996-2014. Ranitidine, Zantac: Drug Facts, Side Effects and Dosing. [Online] Available at: http://www.medicinenet.com/ranitidine/article.htm [Accessed 17 March 2014].

38. Heal Pharmacy, Zantac (Ranitidine) generic [Online] Available at http://www.healpharmacy.com/zantac-ranitidine-150-032-180-pills-p-5472.html. [Accessed Feb 2015]

39. Zoom Info, Dr. Jeffrey Phillips, Research Associate professor, University of Missouri-Columbia, [Online] Available at http://www.zoominfo.com/p/Jeffrey-Phillips/81631039. [Accessed Feb 2015]

40. Infant Acid Reflux Solutions, TummyCare Max and BellyBuffers [Online] Available at: http://www.infant-acid-reflux-solutions.com [Accessed Feb 2015]

41. Smith A. MD, Proton Pump Inhibitors and Clostridium Difficile Infection, March 20, 2014. [Online] Available at: http://www.clinicalcorrelations.org/?p=7409. [Accessed Feb 2015]

42. Woelle, D. K., 2011, the official website of Doctor Kurt Woelle. [Online] Available at: http://drwoeller.com/ [Accessed 20 May 2014].

43. Healthline Networks, Inc., 2005-2014. *Pro-kinetic Agents: Bethanechol, Cisapride, Domperidone, and Metoclopramide.* [Online] Available at: http://www.healthline.com/health/gerd/prokinetics#2 [Accessed 21 June 2014].

44. MedicineNet, Inc., 1996-2014. *Metoclopramide, Reglan: Drug Facts, Side Effects and Dosing.* [Online] Available at: http://www.medicinenet.com/metoclopramide/article.htm [Accessed 30 June 2014].

45. Baxter Healthcare Corporation, n.d. *MEDICATION GUIDE REGLAN (Reg-lan) (metoclopramide) injection,* Deerfield, IL 60015 USA: Baxter Healthcare Corporation.

46. PaddockPhD,Catharine[http://www.medicalnewstoday.com/articles/159914.php] para 5 [Accessed 05 May 2015].

47. GI for Kids, PLLC, 2003-2014. Paediatric Gastroenterology - Barrett's Esophagus - Diseases - East Tennessee Children's Hospital - GI for Kids, PLLC. [Online] Available at: http://www.giforkids.com/?a=Diseases&b=Barrett%27s%20Esophagus [Accessed 09 June 2014].

48. Jolene Beatson, S. W., n.d. *CMPA Support.* [Online] Available at: http://cowsmilkproteinallergysupport.webs.com/ [Accessed 17 June 2014].

49. Ketomi Distribution, Colic Calm @2013-2014. Colic Calm. [Online] Available at: http://www.coliccalm.com.au/blog/cat/baby-colic-gas-reflux [Accessed 12 April 2014].

50. GI for Kids, PLLC, 2003-2014. Paediatric Gastroenterology - Barrett's Esophagus - Diseases - East Tennessee Children's Hospital - GI for Kids, PLLC. [Online] Available at: http://www.giforkids.com/?a=Diseases&b=Barrett%27s%20Esophagus [Accessed 09 June 2014].

51. Kids with Food Allergies, Inc., 2005-2011. *FPIES: Food Protein Induced enterocolitis Syndrome.* [Online] Available at: http://www.kidswithfoodallergies.org/resourcespre.php?id=99# [Accessed 17 June 2014].

52. Info available online. Available at http://labtestsonline.org/understanding/analytes/calprotectin/tab/test. Accessed Mar 2015

53. Trends in Hospitalizations of Children With Inflammatory Bowel Disease Within the United States From 2000 to 2009. Journal of Investigative Medicine, 2013 DOI:10.231/JIM.0b013e31829a4e25

54. Poullis A, Foster R, Mendall MA, Shreeve D, Wiener K (2003). "Proton pump inhibitors are associated with elevation of faecal calprotectin and may affect specificity". Eur J Gastroenterol Hepatol 15(5): 573–4; author reply 574. doi:10.1097/00042737-200305000-00021. PMID 12702920.

55. MARCI-Kids.com, 2007. EXTRA ESOPHAGEAL REFLUX AND SYMPTOMS OF THE EAR, NOSE, THROAT. [Online] Available at http://web.archive.org/web/20081012221121/http://www.marci-kids.com/eerintro.html [Accessed 21 May 2014].

56. For more information and to access the list of references indexed in the above excerpt please use this link: http://web.archive.org/web/20081120220009/http://www.marci-kids.com/eerreferences.html#19

57. Pegeen Eslami, M. A. P. o. P. D. o. P. E. M. U. M. M. C., 1994-2014 . *Sandifer's Syndrome Clinical Presentation.* [Online] Available at: http://emedicine.medscape.com/article/931761-clinical [Accessed 24 May 2014].

58. Jones Dr Fiona , On Call Children's Therapy Network, Suite 6, Leve1 1 Kenmore Village, Kenmore, Queensland, Australia) Phone: 07 3378 9543, Fax: 07 3878 5144 Email: admin@occtherapy.com.au Postal Address: PO Box 1118, Kenmore QLD 4069

59. http://www.citizensinformation.ie/en/employment/employment_rights_and_conditions/leave_and_holidays/maternity_leave.html

60. http://www.citizensinformation.ie/en/employment/employment_rights_and_conditions/leave_and_holidays/parental_leave.html

61. http://www.citizensinformation.ie/en/employment/employment_rights_and_conditions/leave_and_holidays/parental_leave.html

62. http://www.citizensinformation.ie/en/employment/employment_rights_and_conditions/leave_and_holidays/parental_leave.html

63. http://www.citizensinformation.ie/en/employment/employment_rights_and_conditions/leave_and_holidays/parental_leave.html

64. http://www.citizensinformation.ie/en/employment/employment_rights_and_conditions/leave_and_holidays/parental_leave.html

Appendix 1

MARCI Kids Medical References

1. Rosbe KW, Kenna M, Auerbach AD. Extraesophageal reflux in paediatric patients with upper respiratory symptoms. Arch Otolaryngology Head Neck Surg. 2003; 129:1213-1220.

2. DeVault KR. Extraesophageal symptoms of GERD. Cleve Clin J Med. 2003;70(suppl 5):S20-S32.

3. Nelson S, Chen E, Syniar G, Christoffel K. Prevalence of symptoms of gastroesophageal reflux during infancy: a paediatric practice-based survey. Arch Pediatr Adolesc Med. 1997;151:569-572.

4. Little JP, Matthews BL, Glock MS, et al. Extraesophageal paediatric reflux: 24-hour double-probe pH monitoring of 222 children. Ann Otol Rhinol Laryngol. 1997;169 (suppl.):1-16.

5. Mathews BL, Little JP, McGuirt WF Jr, Koufman JA. Reflux in infants with laryngomalacia: results of 24-hour double-probe pH monitoring. Otolaryngol Head Neck Surg. 1999;120:860-864.

6. Bothwell MR, Phillips J, Bauer S. Upper esophageal pH monitoring of children with the Bravo pH capsule. Laryngoscope. 2004;114:786-788.

7. Irwin RS, Boulet LP, Cloutier MM, et al. Managing cough as a defense mechanism and as a symptom:a consensus panel report of the American College of Chest Physicians. Chest. 1998;114(2 Suppl Managing):133S-181S.

8. Holinger LD and Sanders A.D. Chronic cough in infants and children: an update. Laryngoscope. 1991;101: 596-605.

9. Bluestone, CD, Stool S, Kenna, M, et al., ed. Pediatric Otolaryngology. 4th ed. Philadelphia:Saunders; 2003.

10. Kalach, N, Gumpert L, Contencin P, Dupont C. Dual-probe pH monitoring for the assessment of gastroesophageal reflux in the course of chronic hoarseness in children. Turk J Pediatr. 2000; 42:186-91.

11. Powell DM, Karanfilov BI, Beechler KB, Treole K, Trudeau MD, Forrest LA. Paradoxical vocal cord dysfunction in juveniles. Arch Otolaryngol Head Neck Surg. 2000;126: 29-34.

12. Heatley DG, Swift E. Paradoxical vocal cord dysfunction in an infant with stridor and gastroesophageal reflux. Int J Pediatr Otorhinolaryngol. 1996;34:149-151.

13. Hollinger LD. Etiology of stridor in the neonate, infant, and child. Ann Otol Rhinol Larygnol. 1980;89:397-400.

14. Belmont JR, Grundfast K. Congenital laryngeal stridor (laryngomalacia): etiologic factors and associated disorders.Ann Otol Rhinol Laryngol. 1984;93: 430-437.

15. Giannoni C, Sulek M, Friedman, EM. Duncan NO 3rd. Gastroesophageal reflux association with laryngomalacia: a prospective study. Int J Pediatr Otorhinolaryngol. 1998;43:11-20.

16. Little FB, Koufman JA, Kohut RI, Marshall RB. Effect of gastric acid on the pathogenesis of subglottic stenosis. Ann Otol Rhinol Laryngol. 1985;94:516- 519.

17. Waki EY, Madgy DN, Belenky WM, Gower VC. The incidence of gastroesophageal reflux in recurrent croup. Int J Pediatr Otorhinolaryngol. 1995;32:223-32.

18. Yellon R, Parameswaran M, Brandom B. Decreasing morbidity following layrngotracheal reconstruction in children.Int J Ped Otorhinolaryngol. 1997;41:145-154.

19. Halstead LA. Role of gastroesophageal reflux in pediatric upper airway disorders. Otolaryngol Head Neck Surg.1999;120:208-214

20. Halstead LA. Gastroesophageal reflux: a critical factor in pediatric subglottic stenosis. Otolaryngol Head Neck Surg. 1999;120:683-688.

21. Carr MM, Poje CP, Ehrig D, Brodsky LS. Incidence of reflux in young children undergoing adenoidectomy. Laryngoscope. 2001;111:2170-2172.

22. Loehrl TA, Smith TL. Chronic sinusitis and gastroesophageal reflux: are they related? Curr Opin Otolaryngol Head Neck Surg. 2004;12:18-20.

23. Bothwell MR, Parsons DS, Talbot A, Barbero GJ, Wilder B. Outcome of reflux therapy on pediatric chronic sinusitis.Otolaryngol Head Neck Surg. 1999;121:255-62.

24. White DR, Heavner SB, Hardy SM, Prazma J. Gastroesophageal reflux and eustachian tube dysfunction in an animal model. Laryngoscope. 2002;112: 955-61.

25. Heavner SB, Hardy SM, White DR, McQueen CT. Prazma J. Pillsbury HC 3rd. Function of the eustachian tube after weekly exposure to pepsin/hydrochloric acid. Otolaryngol Head Neck Surg. 2001;125:123-129.

26. Poelmans J, Tack J, Feenstra L. Prospective study on the incidence of chronic ear complaints related to gastroesophageal reflux and on the outcome of antireflux therapy. Ann Otol Rhinol Laryngol. 2002;111:933-938.

Lightning Source UK Ltd.
Milton Keynes UK
UKHW021006140819
347957UK00013B/1369/P